Dr Alan H[...] [...] authority o[...] disease from [...] and has edit[...] [...]ooks and published over 200 papers on these subjects. He founded and served as editor of the *International Journal of Obesity* from 1977 to 1983 and is Chairman of the Food Education Society.

Dr Howard received his academic degrees (M.A. and Ph.D) from Cambridge University, and is a Fellow of the Royal Institute of Chemistry. He has served on the Scientific Staff of the Medical Research Council and now works at the Department of Medicine, University of Cambridge, where he is a lecturer on Nutritional Research.

In 1973 Dr Howard collaborated with BBC-TV and participated in its ten part series, 'Don't Just Sit There', designed to motivate people in weight loss.

The Cambridge Diet

Alan Howard

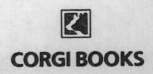

CORGI BOOKS

To Ian McLean Baird, M.D., F.R.C.P.

THE CAMBRIDGE DIET
A CORGI BOOK 0 552 12797 3

Originally published in Great Britain by Jonathan Cape Ltd.

PRINTING HISTORY
Jonathan Cape edition published 1985
Corgi edition published 1986

This book is set in 10/11 pt Baskerville

Corgi Books are published by Transworld Publishers Ltd.,
61-63 Uxbridge Road, Ealing, London W5 5SA,
in Australia by Transworld Publishers (Aust.) Pty. Ltd.,
26 Harley Crescent, Condell Park, NSW 2200, and in New
Zealand by Transworld Publishers (N.Z.) Ltd., Cnr. Moselle
and Waipareira Avenues, Henderson, Auckland.

Made and printed in Great Britain by
Hunt Barnard Printing Ltd., Aylesbury, Bucks.

Contents

Medical Precautions

As with any weight-loss programme, it is recommended that you consult your doctor before commencing the Cambridge Diet. Medical supervision is particularly important when losing weight for the very elderly, growing children and adolescents, or if you have heart and cardiovascular conditions, diabetes, gout, kidney disease, stroke, chronic infections, hypoglycaemia, or are under medical care for any other condition. Your doctor will be able to advise you whether or not you should be on this or any other diet and may want to adjust any medication you are taking. The Cambridge Diet induces water loss when taken as the sole source of nutrition. Therefore, diuretics or any medications which produce water loss should not be taken whilst on the diet, except with the approval of your doctor.

It is unadvisable for pregnant or nursing women or children below twelve years of age to use the Cambridge Diet as a sole source of nutrition. However, all persons may use the Cambridge Diet as a nutritional supplement.

The Cambridge Diet should not be used as the sole source of nutrition for more than four consecutive weeks at any one time unless the patient is under medical supervision.

FOREWORD

Sir John Butterfield, MD, FRCP
Regius Professor of Physic, Cambridge University

I have known Alan Howard for twenty years as a very energetic biochemist and nutritionist. We first became acquainted through our shared research interests. He was particularly concerned about obese people, and at that time I and my colleagues at Guy's Hospital, in London, were looking into the adult onset of diabetes in patients who are usually overweight. For example, why would glucose not move from the blood of ordinary fat people into their muscles (unless they exercised) as it did in thin people? In a way we were finding that almost all fat people were partially diabetic.

Alan Howard's approach to all this was more straight-forward, more practical and much more directly concerned with doing something about the obesity. Quite simply, he wanted to find out the best way to help people become thin, and so he set to work along these lines in the Department of Medicine at Cambridge.

Early on, he was interested in what he called the 'Cambridge Loaf', from which much of the carbo-hydrate had been extracted before the flour was used to make the dough. Then he began to see that it was important not only to provide a low calorie diet but one which also ensured that the dieter would not go without vitamins, minerals or trace elements. He wanted a diet which, if possible, would not turn the body's defences to retaining water and so hinder weight loss. In due course, his clinical colleagues joined in the work and it became clear that their new formula, based on fortified skimmed milk powder, could help people lose weight in a satisfactory way. And it was soon appreciated that the diet had to be so tasty that people really looked forward to taking it, rather than dreading it.

This is the background to the story which Alan Howard has set out in his book. Of course, there have been ups and downs in his adventures, while he searched for an ideal weight-reducing diet. He faced problems trying to find a British firm to follow his lead, and then ran into difficulties with some critical members of the medical profession in the USA. Pioneers in these things never have an easy or instant success, especially in a field like weight reduction. Yet Alan's personal sense of purpose, of urgency, and his genuine concern for overweight people, individuals who need his skills and ideas and his persuasion in order to help themselves, all come over strongly in these pages.

Here then is the story of an exceptional scientist, who has shown perseverance in this basic research work and persistence in his efforts to develop his ideas with a view to helping not only a very large number of overweight people but, maybe soon, other categories of patients as well. I will be surprised if the reader of this fascinating book is not gripped by its account of his efforts so far, and its presentation of ideas he is developing for the future.

PREFACE

The Cambridge Diet arose out of more than eight years of research and development at the University of Cambridge and the West Middlesex Hospital, London. The formula contains only 330 calories but is otherwise complete in all essential nutrients. Overweight people are advised to follow the diet as the sole source of nutrition; without any additional food, substantial weight losses, approaching those seen in complete starvation, can be readily achieved with absolute safety.

Many overweight people have had their lives beneficially changed by using the Cambridge Diet, and to illustrate its value I have included a number of personal stories. All the people really exist and their actual names have been used.

The Cambridge Diet was first introduced to the United States in the spring of 1980. Because it is relatively new to Europe, one purpose of this book is to acquaint the public with the principles behind the diet and to tell the story of its research and development.

Since 1981 the Cambridge Diet has been distributed through a new system of agents called 'Cambridge Counsellors'. These are people who had benefited from using the diet and wished to communicate their experience to others. By mid-1982 there were 200,000 Counsellors and regular users in excess of three million people.

Despite its obvious success and public usefulness, the diet then came under fierce attack from a number of obesity experts in the medical establishment. At first it was maintained that the diet's formulation was contrary to recognized nutritional principles, and its low protein and caloric content harmful. Later on the experts admitted the diet was effective but insisted that it should be used only under supervision 'in selected clinics and university medical schools, specializing in such treatment'.

However, in the world outside their university hospitals, the situation was quite different. Hundreds of general practitioners and some other university doctors found that their patients experienced very substantial weight losses, with few or no side effects. To them, the diet looked very benign and safe.

Against this background of controversy I decided that now is the appropriate time to write a book about the Cambridge Diet, not only to explain how and why it is effective, but also to dispel many of the misconceptions that have arisen about it. My viewpoint is that any new principle in science is bound to cause debate and to arouse controversy.

The Cambridge Diet was originally intended as a formulation for weight loss, but in my opinion great value lies in its use as a nutritious food to provide a daily baseline intake of essential nutrients, both in the developed nations and in the Third World. I believe this aspect of the use of the Cambridge Diet may be one of its most important functions for the future, and I have discussed this subject in the book accordingly.

Cambridge   A.H.
1985

Further information about the availability of the diet can be obtained from:

CAMBRIDGE NUTRITION LIMITED,
69-75 THORPE ROAD,
NORWICH,
NORFOLK NR1 1HY.

ACKNOWLEDGEMENTS

Many people have helped me to write this book. I must gratefully thank Eleanor Harnish from Norman, Oklahoma, for compiling information, interviewing successful dieters and recording their stories, and expertly manipulating the word processor; my secretary, Mary Miller, for typing, and Rita Steffensen for advising on the literary style, and members of my family and others who read the manuscript and made valuable suggestions. I also wish to thank Sheila and Dennis Ignasias and Slim-lines Publications of Salisbury, Maryland, USA, for permission to reproduce extracts from their booklet, *Recipes for use with the Cambridge Diet*, 1983, and Metropolitan Life Insurance Co. for permission to reproduce the height and weight tables in Appendix 2.

Writing this book also gives me the opportunity to thank all those who participated in the development and clinical trials of the Cambridge Diet. Among the foremost of these is Dr Ian McLean Baird, to whom this book is dedicated and without whom the work could never have been accomplished; Professor Sir John Butterfield, head of the Clinical School, University of Cambridge, for his interest and moral support; Professor Ivor Mills for allowing the work to take place in his department and for constant encouragement. Among the doctors who supervised the Obesity Clinic at Addenbrooke's Hospital were Andrew Grant, Ray Moore, Russell Cook, Steve Olczak, John Marks, Andrew Brooks, Huw Alban Davies. Technical assistance was given by Michael and Betty Brown, Aileen

Bright, and Shashi Rattan. At the West Middlesex Hospital, the doctors included Ray Parsons and E.R. Littlewood. The project could never have succeeded without the untiring devotion of Mrs Joan Fowler, who was in charge of the day-to-day handling of the inpatients at the West Middlesex Hospital. On the commercial side, I am especially indebted to Dr Dennis Jones, formerly of Organon, without whose help the Diet certainly would never have been made accessible to the public; also to Jack, Eileen and Vaughn Feather, of Monterey, California, who had the foresight to see its great potential.

PART 1

The Cambridge Plan

CHAPTER ONE

THE PERFECT DIET

Newspapers and magazines are full of articles about slimming. 'Lose 5 lbs (2 kg) In Five Days' is the sort of headline frequently seen in our Sunday newspapers. It seems that very many people are obsessed with losing weight. Why should there be so much fuss about it when everybody knows that the only effective way to reduce is to eat less?

Dieting is by no means an easy undertaking. In fact it is extremely difficult. Mark Twain's remark about smoking – 'It's easy to give up, I've done it many times' – is equally true of slimming.

There are innumerable systems of dieting in existence. There is even an encyclopedia of diets available which lists 200 new diets, and even these do not include the Scarsdale, Atkins, Beverly Hills or the F-Plan diets. Those who follow any one of these diets will almost certainly lose weight. The first 5 lbs (2 kg) will fall off easily, but what then?

People approach dieting in different ways, but a number of generalizations can be made. When it comes to giving up eating, most of us are only willing to make sacrifices for a short time. We like food. It is easy to take, and very pleasurable. Dieting is inconvenient. It interferes with parties, business lunches, holidays, and makes one feel a social outcast.

For most people the perfect diet should guarantee rapid loss of weight, so that a resumption of eating whatever is considered to be 'Real Food' may be delayed for as short a time as possible.

Why Diets Fail

Despite the warnings of experts, who maintain that crash diets are dangerous, these are precisely what the ordinary overweight man or woman wants. Unfortunately crash diets *are* usually dangerous (though not always) and have unpleasant side effects. Some rely on a confidence trick in which water is simply lost instead of fat. Those who try them often end up feeling very sceptical and still overweight.

The chief dieting season is in the spring, before the annual jaunt to the beach, where great embarrassment may be caused by one's excessive corpulence. Many people are prepared to diet for a month or two then and attempt to follow the latest diet seen in a magazine or newspaper. Initially they are delighted with the loss of 5-10 lbs (2-4 kg). Then after a few weeks a plateau is reached and nothing further seems to happen. The weight comes off very slowly, or not at all, and the would-be slimmers give up.

Although still overweight, these people will have lost just enough weight to allow them to believe the result worthwhile. The real reason for discontinuing is the fact that they get stuck. If the weight loss continued then many people would go on and on until they achieved their ideal body weight. What happens next? The average dieter goes back to normal eating and in almost the same length of time, four to six weeks, without apparently over-indulging, is back to exactly what he or she weighed before.

So the process goes on from year to year. In early spring there is the desire to lose weight and attempt a new diet; in the summer, complete failure and the realization that there seems very little one can do but remain fat.

The reason for this yo-yo effect is not altogether clear, but there are clues to its cause. The individual weight tends to oscillate around what is called a set-point. If you overindulge when you are thin, or go on a diet when you are fat, you always return to approximately the same weight – your set-point. Whatever dietary manoeuvres you adopt you will eventually return to it. The set-point can be changed, particularly upwards, over the course of time and may be considerably higher at the age of 50 than it was when you were 30. It is controlled principally by your metabolic rate and your appetite.

When people go on a slimming diet and reduce their calorie intake, the metabolic rate falls, which simply means that less energy than before is needed to maintain body weight. Someone eating about 2,500 calories a day, who then reduces the daily intake to 1,000 calories, will experience an encouraging weight loss in the first one or two weeks. At the end of four weeks the metabolic rate will fall and the body adjust to the new 1,000 calorie intake so that there is little further weight-loss.

It is this downward change in metabolic rate which explains why dieters put on weight easily after resuming their normal food consumption. With a lower metabolic rate after dieting, an increase of calories provides more than sufficient energy to maintain body weight, and the excess goes to produce a weight increase. Weight will be gained very rapidly in succeeding weeks, and may even go higher than it was before dieting. The idea that dieting makes you fat has considerable truth in it.

What exactly controls the metabolic rate and the set-point is very complex and currently the subject of a great deal of research in medical schools throughout the world. Basically, it is believed that the activity of the thyroid and adrenal hormones falls during dieting, and that this is responsible for the fall in energy output. After resumption of normal eating it takes time for the body to readjust. Much of the food eaten is not utilized for energy and so becomes converted to body fat.

Another important factor in the process of regaining weight is appetite. After a diet people often feel more hungry than usual, and, without the mental constraint of dieting, they eat more. Control of appetite is probably also affected by hormones, particularly those which are released into the stomach and intestines and become absorbed into the blood stream, so signalling to the brain that we should eat more.

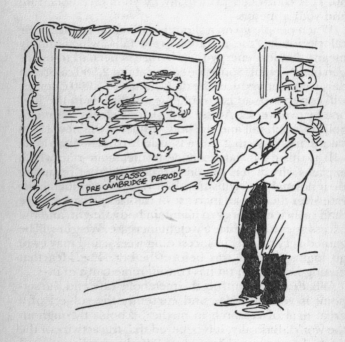

The effect of weight loss on both the metabolic rate and the appetite is geared to regain all the weight we have lost. To our ancestors, being fat was considered beneficial to survival. The fat man lived longer because he carried around his own energy reserves in the form of body fat. During periods of famine the metabolic rate decreased so as to minimize energy loss. When food became plentiful again, both metabolism and appetite were set so as to regain the weight lost as quickly as possible. In our industrialized society we continue to protect ourselves, unnecessarily, in this way. What was advantageous to our forebears ends up as a great hindrance to those of us who wish to appear slim and enjoy many years of healthy life.

The Cambridge Diet Explained

So what is the perfect diet? It is one that works quickly and produces excellent weight loss in the shortest poss-ible time. For most people this means within a few weeks or, at the most, two or three months, to obtain their ideal body weight. It should be easy, relatively inexpensive, nutritious and healthy, have no or few side effects and be fundamentally safe. More important still, the diet should enable one to maintain the body weight after dieting and to resist the yo-yo effect and the desire of the body to regain its previous set-point. I believe that the Cambridge Diet fulfils all these requirements.

The Cambridge Diet is a nutritionally complete for-mula which contains only 330 calories per day. No one can fail to lose weight consistently on so few calories. It is a near starvation diet and yet supplies all the essential nutrients the body needs. An overweight person follow-ing the diet lives on his or her body fat just like a camel. So long as there is body fat available to provide energy the dieter will lose weight safely and surely!

By any standards the weight losses achievable through the Cambridge Diet are exceptional: an average of 18 lbs (8 kg) in four weeks, and about 14 lbs (6 kg) in each month thereafter. It is common for people on the Cambridge Diet to lose a total of 70 to 100 lbs (31.75-44.45 kg), and the record weight loss is 25 stone (350 lbs; 158.75 kg). Such losses are very close to what might be expected from complete starvation – the so-called 'Zero Calorie Diet'. Without any food at all in his diet, a man would lose 20 lbs (9 kg) instead of the 18 lbs (8 kg) each month on the Cambridge Diet. Thus the Cambridge Diet provides the most rapid weight loss consistent with good health and well-being.

The diet is very easy and pleasant to take and comes in a number of different guises – soups, milk-shakes, desserts, each portion containing about 110 calories. To lose weight the dieter consumes three portions of diet each day, using any one of these different varieties, together with plenty of water. Very few slimmers suffer from menu fatigue when on the Cambridge Diet since there are six varieties of soups and five drinks. However, some slimmers miss the opportunity to chew. For this reason, a range of Cambridge Diet Meal Replacement Bars have been developed. Designed along the same lines as the Cambridge Diet, each meal bar contains a precise balance of protein, carbohydrate, fat, vitamins and minerals and even though coated with milk chocolate contains only 140 calories per bar. Each bar weighs 55 grams and contains 11 grams of dietary fibre, which is approximately one third of the intake advised by nutritionists. The five flavours include Toffee, Peanut, Chocolate, Lemon and Ginger and Caramel. The only other foods allowed are black coffee, tea and calorie-free drinks. This use of the Cambridge Diet as the sole source of nutrition can be followed for periods of up to a month, and even longer if under the care of a doctor. If further weight loss is required the diet should be supplemented, for one week, with food of about 400 calories a day, before returning to the unsupplemented diet again.

The Cambridge Diet is not available at chemists or supermarkets, but is sold only through independent members of the public known as 'Cambridge Counsellors'. These people have benefited previously by losing weight themselves, or else use the diet as a nutritional supplement. Their main purpose is to inspire others to emulate their own slimming success, to see the diet is used correctly, to offer support and encouragement and to answer questions. The Cambridge Counsellor is trained and will organize Cambridge Meetings at which potential dieters can obtain information and are introduced to a new life-style.

This method of distribution, introduced several years ago in the United States, is ideal for this type of diet. Without encouragement it is difficult for any one to embark on such a very low calorie diet. If the diet were available on the shelves of chemists, few would have the motivation necessary to keep to it for more than a day or so.

After achieving an ideal weight, it is then possible to reach a new and lower set-point, and to counteract the effects of the yo-yo syndrome. It is here that the Cambridge Diet is most successful. Once off the diet as sole food, the dieter will continue taking the Cambridge Diet three times a day and supplement it with ordinary food of modest calorie content. One balanced meal of about 400 calories each day is recommended. Gradually the ordinary food intake can be increased until weight is maintained at a new set-point – the ideal weight. If social or business life interferes too much with this regime and too many calories are consumed, then the patron simply goes back to the diet as sole source for a few days.

Before the advent of the Cambridge Diet, there was no nutritional regime which could promise permanent weight reduction. Statistics compiled through the help of Cambridge Counsellors have established that 60 per cent of people who lose a substantial amount of weight and who continue to use the Cambridge Diet, are able successfully to keep their excess weight off.

Is it Safe?

It should be emphasised that this is not a 'fad diet'. Before marketing, eight years of research work went into its development and already it has been used successfully by large numbers of severely overweight people for long periods of time. Research on the diet started in 1970 at the West Middlesex Hospital, London, when Dr Ian McLean Baird and I decided to collaborate on the development of a new formula diet which could contain the fewest calories consistent with safety and good health.

Many of the popular diets recommended in magazines have very little scientific basis and certainly few have been tested in clinical trials. Both Dr Baird and I felt very strongly that before the Cambridge Diet was 'unleashed' on the general public, it should undergo the most rigorous testing, especially to establish its safety. We knew there would be scepticism and our professional reputations were at stake.

The diet was tested in much the same way as a new drug is. Many routine tests were conducted on hundreds of patients over long periods. No side effects of any major concern were encountered, and at the end of many years of study it was pronounced safe.

During the clinical trials, the Cambridge Diet was found to confer a number of distinct advantages. Among these were a decrease in blood fats and a lowering of blood pressure which in turn reduced the risk of coronary heart disease and strokes. The diet was also found to be very suitable for overweight diabetics, although it is important for a doctor to discontinue or adjust their usual medication.

Since it is not possible to devise a diet from natural foodstuffs containing all the nutrients a person needs in just 330 calories, the Cambridge Diet has to be made as a formulation in which vitamins, minerals and trace elements are added. In order to make it palatable, flavours are introduced so as to simulate natural foods and promote enjoyment. In the broadest sense, the diet is a summation of all the research on nutrition and food technology of this century and brings the work of hundreds of thousands of scientists and doctors to fruition. Before it could be manufactured, our knowledge had to advance to the stage where all important vitamins, minerals and trace elements were identified and could be produced inexpensively and in large quantities. It is only in the last few years that this has become possible. That is why the Cambridge Diet (or something resembling it) has not evolved until quite recently. It was technically impossible!

Besides the extensive use of the Cambridge Diet for weight maintenance, many people – especially athletes – find it beneficial as a nutritional supplement, even where being over-weight has never been a problem. Its regular consumption in the United States and Europe by hundreds of thousands of people for this purpose has established the Cambridge Diet as a staple foodstuff with many advantages. It is the most nutritionally dense food that exists, and contains all the basic nutrients, except calories, required by man.

For Better Health

In a civilization relying so much on manufactured and 'fast foods' (which are highly refined and often almost devoid of nutritional value), I believe such a complete foodstuff is needed to ensure adequate and balanced nutrition for those who are interested in obtaining it. Many expert nutritionists disagree with this view and instead they advocate eating a wide selection of different types of food – what they call eating 'sensibly' – so as to include all the different nutrients in the correct amount we need. If people have the skill to plan their diet well, this can indeed be accomplished relatively

23

easily and inexpensively. Few, however, devote the necessary time to such an important subject. How many people know how much zinc or copper they consumed yesterday, or today, or will consume tomorrow? To calculate the whole range of important nutrients in the foods you have eaten would take many hours – even using a computer.

From time to time, nutritional surveys are conducted into what various groups of people in the population – such as children, pregnant women, the elderly and minority ethnic groups – actually eat. The usual story is that there is some nutrient which is not being taken in adequate amounts. It may be vitamin C or A, or iron or copper. Very often it is found that different groups of people have different deficiencies, and that it is important for them to know what supplement or additional types of food they should be eating for perfect health. By consuming a complete foodstuff, like the Cambridge Diet, anyone can be sure that every nutrient is taken, in just the right amount, every day.

It is usual for people losing weight on the Cambridge Diet to remark on how much better they feel. Of course, a lot of the benefit can be accounted for by their loss of weight. But it is equally due to the improvement in nutrition. Overweight people very often eat the wrong foods and are malnourished. Perhaps for the first time in their lives they are consuming the perfect food and understandably feel the benefit. Consequently they usually wish to continue with the diet as a nutritional supplement even after their ideal weight has been reached.

It is hoped that the Cambridge Diet will make a major contribution towards the health of the nation, especially if it is combined with other changes in our eating habits. Government authorities now recommend that we eat fewer animal fats and less salt and sugar, and that we consume more fibre. By so doing, the incidence of complaints such as coronary heart disease, stroke,

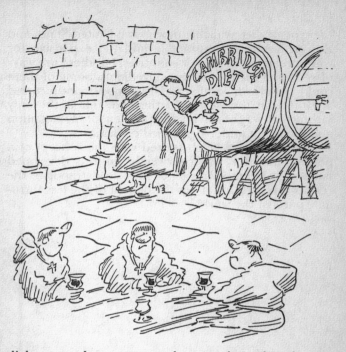

diabetes and cancer can be greatly reduced. The Cambridge Counsellor makes a major contribution by drawing attention to these facts. A combination of the Cambridge Diet and sound nutritional principles could have a synergistic effect, and lead to many people living longer and healthier lives.

Besides being nutritious, the Cambridge Diet formulation can be made very stable, and so has considerable potential use in the Third World, both as an item of food for storage in case of famine, and also as a staple food to ensure adequate nutrition. Although research in this area is still very much in its infancy, discussions with American scientists, who are establishing the ground-work for the substantial programme needed to develop this aspect, have already taken place. Obviously, the type of diet available now in the United States and Europe would be unsuitable and too expensive for widespread use in poorer countries, but there are ways of reducing the cost of the ingredients. Some of them could be grown locally and the food manufactured anywhere in the world. In the end, this is the only satisfactory way of solving the problem of malnutrition and famine in under-developed countries.

From a project which started with the concept of a perfect diet for the overweight in the developed nations, it is gratifying to be able to extrapolate the results achieved so far for the benefit of the less fortunate parts of the world.

CHAPTER TWO

THE MOTIVATION OF SUCCESS

Motivation

No overweight person can ever succeed on the Cambridge Diet unless he or she is strongly motivated. Just to start requires a positive decision to give up eating food and consume only the Cambridge Diet three times a day. Millions have done it, but can you? Most people will take a hard look at what they are going to gain. Will they really lose weight quickly and will the fat roll off as the weeks go by? Having struggled valiantly and succeeded in reaching their ideal weight, can they maintain it?

At a Cambridge Meeting it is standard procedure for those who have succeeded to come forward and tell of their experiences, rather like a convert at a 'hot gospel meeting'. Nothing can be more motivating than to hear from the lips of someone who has been successful with the diet and to learn how it has changed their lives.

In a book you cannot meet people in person and I can only relate some of the success stories, which are typical of many. It is better to hear and see the person concerned but you may find the following accounts quite stimulating. These people actually exist and their real names are used. I am quoting from their lips with a minimum of editing, and I hope you will find these success stories helpful in motivating you.

Personal Story of Beverley Gordon, Downham Market, Norfolk

'Since about the age of 7 I have always been fat. My mum was working on the farm and so I stayed with my grandmother after school. Being old fashioned she would worry that I hadn't eaten enough and would make me tea with sandwiches and cakes. Then I would go home and have a cooked tea there. Often I would go to the neighbours and they'd heap my plate up with a third tea of chips. I just kept gaining weight.

'At Primary school the other children didn't seem to notice my weight as I just slowly began putting it on, but when I got to Comprehensive school it was different. They didn't know me there and I was called "Billy Bunter", "Fatty" and "Slim" (I don't mind being called "Slim" now).

'It was absolutely disgusting. I felt big and bulky, and didn't want to do anything. I would just sit around and do nothing. When friends and I went to the pictures I would squeeze into one side of the seat and then wiggle about and put the other side in. After the pictures I would suggest we go get something to eat. If my friends had one chocolate bar, I would have two.

'What finally made me do something about my weight was my brother's job. He is a hairdresser and would get into hair fashion shows using models. I wanted so much to be one of his models, to be on stage, parading around and showing how beautiful my hair was. But at 16 stone he wouldn't ask me to be up there with 250 people watching!

'My brother is on his feet all day long and has to bend over a lot. He began to have a bad back. As he had gained about ½ a stone he decided to go on the Cambrdge Diet. When his Cambridge Counsellor came into the shop to get her hair done he told her about me, and so on the 29th of December 1984 I started the diet. I really had no problems at all. It was easy for me –

28

when I'd come down the stairs in the morning I would just tell the family to get my Cambridge Diet ready quickly so I wouldn't want to eat. It only took me 4 months to lose 6 stone, and reach my goal weight of under 10 stone.

'I lost weight where I needed to so that my figure is not only slimmer but is better proportioned. I lost 20 in. from my hips, 15 in. from my waist and only 8 in. from my bust. My life is completely changed. Before I could never have gone to a disco. All my clothes were ugly and old fashioned with huge flowers because that was all I could buy in my store. I felt very old. Now I wear smart, fashionable clothes and go to disco's and have a boyfriend. When I was fat I couldn't even get a boy to give me a glance!

'Today I do exercises, play squash, go swimming and have a weekend job. In sports at school I even use the trampoline, where before I couldn't even get on one.

I have no problem controlling my weight. I try very hard to eat more nutritiously. I used to eat sweets, fruit cake and puddings and I have now learned to eat healthy salads and more nourishing foods.

'There is a hair fashion show with photographers coming up in April and I hope to be one of the models. I have lots to thank the Cambridge Diet for – a whole new, exciting life.

Personal Story of Olive Patterson, Haverhill, Essex

'I started the diet weighing 280 lbs (20 st.; 127 kg) and now I weigh 130 lbs (9 st. 4 lbs; 59 kg). I lost this weight in eight months on the Cambridge Diet.

'I started putting on weight when I had my first child at age 18 and never was able to take it off after that time.

'I went on myriads of diets, would lose a little and gain it right back. It went on and on and I never ever lost weight permanently.

29

'When I was 53 I looked at myself and said "I've had enough." I had been getting fatter and fatter and was feeling very ill. I couldn't get across the road to the shops or climb up the stairs. It was dreadful. Unless you have ever been terribly fat you wouldn't know or understand.

'So, I went to see my doctor and said "I think it's about time you did something for me." I think that he could see that I was really in the mood to do something for myself, and he sent me to the Obesity Clinic at Addenbrooke's Hospital where I met a very nice doctor and he explained the Cambridge Diet to me and I started.

'In the first week I lost about 8 lbs (3.6 kg). Then in the first month I had lost 2 stone (12.7 kg) and it just kept coming off and I went down and down. From then on I just haven't looked back.

'I was hungry in the beginning, very hungry, but it wasn't a REAL hunger, it was just habit. I would go to the cupboards and look around, put something in my mouth, remember my diet and run to spit it out. I can honestly say, and it's hard to believe, I never cheated once!

'I felt really well on the diet. In fact, I've never felt so well as I have on this diet. I've had no problems. As I like all foods and I really like to eat I was sure I would find it difficult. I expected to have problems, but in fact I felt actually full, and there was no trouble staying on the diet. The motivation of seeing the fat coming off and because I felt so well kept me on the diet.

'Also, the fact that I knew I was getting everything the body needed in the diet, and I did not need to weigh out this or that, count this or that calorie made it easy for me. I just took the Cambridge Diet three times a day and that was it. I just knew I was safe, getting what I needed and it was easy, and it worked!!

'I did exercise, mildly, for about fifteen minutes a day.

'I have kept the weight off for over a year now, continuing on the maintenance programme. I still have the diet twice a day (breakfast and lunch) and eat one regular meal in the evening with my family.

'If I want to go out, or there is a birthday celebration, anniversary or whatever, I enjoy myself and then just go on the diet sole source the following day. I have learned that I cannot eat over 850 calories a day.

'There has never been a time when I let myself slip back into the old ways. When you have been as fat as I was and been as ill as I was, there is no way I would go back.

'My family is absolutely thrilled with the new me. They really are excited. I have lost more than another whole person and have virtually no sagging skin and I don't look haggard.

'If I can ever help anyone else go on this diet I'd be so glad to help them. It has made a new life for me, really.

'There was a time when my husband used to walk behind or in front of me so he could pretend he wasn't with me. He used to have to actually park the car in front of the shop, because I couldn't walk. Now he is very proud of me. It has been unbelievable!

'And what a great time I had buying new clothes! It was such fun. I went from a size 30 to a size 12.

'All I can say is for me it's been a miracle, it really has!'

Olive Patterson is now a Cambridge Counsellor.

Personal Story of Michael Friday, Oxford

I have always had a weight problem. It started when I was about 10 years old. I had played rugger before that and I suppose the exercise kept my weight in control. After I stopped playing the weight began to come on. I got up to 16 stone and then by the age of 24 I weighed a big 20 to 21 stone. I began to diet on just a regular diet of counting calories and watching what I ate. It took me 2½ years to lose 4 stone.

'In 1975 I had a nervous breakdown. I felt dreadful and just lost control of my weight. I was on medication for my depression and it made me feel awful. I shot up to 19 stone again and had very high blood pressure. The doctor put me on tablets for the blood pressure, but I had bought a small business and with the stress and so on, I stopped taking them. I kept gaining even more weight until on February 1985 I was up to 23½ stone. My blood pressure was so high that the doctor told me I would have to go back on medication for the rest of my life. That really made me feel bad and it was at this time that I went on the Cambridge Diet.

'I quickly lost 2 stone. When I went to my doctor and told him I was on the diet he told me to stop taking it for five days. He took a blood sample and I went on home. When I went back five days later he said that my blood contained all the necessary elements that I needed and that there was no sign of anaemia. He then took my blood pressure and found that it had dropped so much that he was greatly encouraged and told me to go back on the Cambridge Diet. I then lost 6 stone more, making it a total weight loss of 8 stone in 14 weeks.

'The interesting thing about my blood pressure is that when I had reached 17 stone the doctor took me completely off all my tablets and I felt so much better. One month later, at 15½ stone, my blood pressure was completely normal and the doctor told me I didn't need to see him again for six months! As I am 6ft. 5½ in. tall he did feel that I was a bit underweight at 15½ stone and suggested that I regain half a stone.

'I own my own business and because of the high blood pressure and my age of 47 years, I had been unable to get life insurance. Once my blood pressure became normal my doctor suggested that I could apply. I went to the insurance company and gave them my medical history. They arranged for a private examination and, at 15 stone 10 and with normal blood pressure, I was issued a life insurance policy without any penalties. My blood pressure was 110/80.

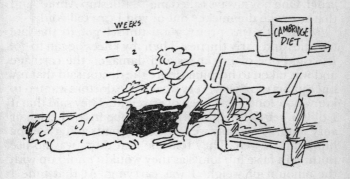

'The great thing about the Cambridge Diet is that I lost weight where it was needed. On other diets my wrists and fingers would get thin. I couldn't even keep a ring on my finger. My waist had been 48 in. and after the Cambridge Diet is now 38 in., my chest was 56 in. and went down to 45 in. I wore a 21 in. collar and can now buy a 17½ shirt.

'I now feel very fit and have a whole new life. I'm even playing squash. It's just fantastic.'

Personal Story of Ann Gibbons, Clacton-on-Sea, Essex

'I've been overweight since the age of nine. By the time I reached thirteen I was a real heavy-weight. No one really seemed to know why, they just said that I was built big. I tried diets with doctors and at hospitals, they were mostly calorie control diets. For the most part doctors couldn't tell me anything or do anything to help me.

'At first they told me it must be the way I ate, but I knew it wasn't that. Things went from bad to worse as I grew older. At school I couldn't run in sports or do PT as the other children did. I would get out of breath, of course, carrying all that weight. And children can be cruel. One boy always called me "Battleship Annie" and that can take the mickey out of you I can tell you!

'My health was pretty good until I got to the late twenties and early thirties. Then my knees began to go. I twisted one of my knees and damaged the cartilage and was taken to hospital where the doctor said that my knee joints were very, very weak. The doctors wanted to know how long I had been overweight. They said that if I didn't get the weight off I would be in a wheelchair very soon, as not only were the knee joints going but the hip joints as well. They told me that there was no use putting in false hip joints as they wouldn't hold up with the amount of weight I was carrying. At that time I weighed 20 stone (280 lbs; 127 kg).

'The doctors then put me under a dietitian at Clacton Hospital and she put me on an 800 calorie diet. It took me 15 months to get off 5 stone (70 lbs; 31.75 kg). During this time I was very ill. I had no energy and fell asleep all the time.

'By the time I got married in 1978 I had gradually gained back weight until I weighed 17 stone (238 lbs; 108 kg). My social life was nil. I was ashamed to go to parties and dances and although my husband was a great walker, I would sit in the car and wait, because I could only walk a few yards as I couldn't breathe, and I would get pains in my chest and legs and my knees hurt.

'I was so miserable and unhappy. At age 39, height 5 ft 1 in. (155 cm), I weighed 21 stone (294 lbs; 133 kg). My hips were 68 in. (173 cm), waist 55 (140 cm) and bust 52 (132 cm). I could no longer wear Evans Outsize largest size (32). I'd fall asleep in my chair at all hours of the day. Everything was too much trouble for me and I was suffering terrible chest pains. My husband finally said I had to do something. He and my step-daughter had seen a programme on BBC TV on Addenbrooke's

34

Hospital about their Obesity Clinic and he thought I should ask my doctor about it.

'On November 5, 1982, I weighed in at Addenbrooke's Hospital. Imagine my chagrin when I found they couldn't weigh me on their chair scale – it didn't go that high! I had to go to another scale and I was humiliated. I was examined and told that I simply had to get the weight off as my heart was showing signs of great strain! I was then given a briefing on taking the Cambridge Diet. And so began the year-long journey that was to change my life!

'Right from the beginning it was exciting. I began to lose weight immediately and it came off so quickly that my mum had to keep taking my clothes in and then in again. (I wouldn't buy anything new until I had reached goal weight – I knew that this time I could do it!)

'We never socialized because I was so heavy and ashamed. But as I began really coming down in weight we started having dinner parties at home. I didn't mind cooking at all and I'd sit at the table with my glass of Cambridge Diet and feel quite proud that I could do it. And when our friends would say, "Oh, Ann, aren't you good. I don't see how you do it!" I would think, "I am good, aren't I?" It gave me a sense of accomplishment and raised my self-esteem. I felt proud that I could do it!

'Then people really began to notice my weight loss. Some would pass me and wouldn't even recognize me. Everyone was astonished! I lost 11 stone (154 lbs; 70 kg) in eleven months, and then went on to lose one more stone (6 kg), which was my target weight loss of 12 stone (168 lbs; 76 kg). I had actually lost another whole person. My hips are now 37 in. (94 cm), waist 29 (73.5 cm) and bust 36 (91 cm).

'While I was attending the clinic they took many tests and discovered that I had an over-efficient metabolism. It was found that I couldn't have over 650 calories a day. I have therefore learned the secret of maintaining my weight loss. I take three Cambridge Diet meals a day; for breakfast and lunch and the third serving about 5 p.m. I then eat a small meal about 6.30 p.m.

'It has definitely changed my life! My family and friends have said that even my personality has changed. I was very shy before and wouldn't have dreamed of talking to anyone the way I do now. [Ann shares her story with many others as she is now a Cambridge Counsellor.] In fact, I have almost become extroverted.

'Now my husband is having fun just keeping up with me. I'm forever after him to take me to dances. I'm buying fitted clothes to show off my waistline now and I love wearing my tight, stretch jeans. Also, I can now walk with my husband and we take the dogs (actually they prefer running to walking) so we run to keep up with them. I get a good bit of exercise now!

'My husband has really benefited the most, though. He married a big, fat lady who could hardly do anything and now he has a wife he can be proud of. (I must admit I cost him a good amount of money to re-build my wardrobe, but he says it's worth it.) I now have three wardrobes of clothes and I know that I'll always be able to wear them – I'll never go back to being fat again. I have the Cambridge Diet. It is the only diet I know that I can safely use to watch my weight. I weigh every day and should I go up a bit I cut right back. I've maintained my weight for three years now, and I know I can do it for ever thanks to the Cambridge Diet!'

CHAPTER THREE

THE VITAL STEPS

What you have learned about the Cambridge Diet so far may have encouraged you to make a start. When you begin the diet the first few weeks will be quite different from anything else you have ever experienced before in your life. So it is important to tackle it in the right way and logically.

Are You Overweight?

Most people know if they are overweight or not just by looking in a full-length mirror. However, as a guide, tables are provided in Appendix 2 to help you decide.

If you weigh more than 10 lbs (4.5 kg) over the figure quoted for your height and build, then you are definitely overweight.

Seeing Your Doctor

It is recommended that you see your doctor before starting the Cambridge Diet. Just tell him that you would like to start the diet and ask him if he can see any reason for not doing so. If he thinks you should not, please ask him why, and assure yourself that it isn't just because he's prejudiced and thinks that anything below 1,000 calories per day is dangerous. Tell him that the Cambridge Diet is a 'very low calorie' diet of 330 calories. Most doctors these days will be acquainted with such a diet and will already have had practical experience. If he is still puzzled, show him a copy of this book or give him one of the leaflets intended for doctors.

There may be very sound reasons why he feels that you should not embark on the Cambridge Diet and you should listen carefully to his advice. If you have any chronic medical condition, your doctor will need to consider if the Cambridge Diet is suitable. These conditions include: *heart* or *cardiovascular conditions, diabetes, gout, kidney disease, stroke, chronic infections,* and *hypoglycemia.* Here are some of the factors he may take into consideration:

1 *Exclusions.* There are certain people who should not use the Cambridge Diet as a sole source of food (although everyone can use it as a nutritional supplement). These are *pregnant* and *nursing women* or *children below the age of twelve.* The reason for these exclusions is that the protein requirements of people in these categories are much higher than normal, and the diet would not supply them with enough of this vital nutrient. However, if your doctor decides that despite these circumstances you should lose weight, then it is possible to use the Cambridge Diet as part of a supervised diet which contains more calories than the Cambridge Diet does on its own. Also to be considered are the *elderly.* Many overweight people in their seventies have lost a great deal of weight on the Cambridge Diet, and age by itself does not debar people from using it. Yet because of their general medical condition, a doctor might recommend that the diet is not taken as the sole source of food but only as a nutritional supplement.

2 *High blood pressure.* If you are taking diuretics for high blood pressure it is most important that the doctor considers your case very carefully. Diuretics

cause a large excretion of potassium. Combined with the Cambridge Diet this can be dangerous, because the loss will then become too excessive. As, however, the Cambridge Diet, sole source, has a favourable effect on blood pressure and causes it to decrease, most doctors are willing to allow you to discontinue diuretics while you are on it exclusively.

If you are on other medication for high blood pressure such as Methyldopa, it may need to be reduced or discontinued.

3 *Diabetes*. If you have diabetes, and are not taking any drugs, but are controlling your diabetes by diet, there are no problems. The diet contains only 45 grams per day of carbohydrate, and it should be possible for you to use it as sole source beneficially. You can discontinue oral medication completely while you are on the diet sole source, if your doctor so advises. However, the situation with insulin is complicated, and your doctor might need to lower the dose and to re-monitor your blood sugar.

4 *Heart conditions*. Many overweight people who have had a heart attack and recovered have managed to lose a great deal of weight through the Cambridge Diet without complications. In your case, the doctor will have to assess the benefits of losing weight against the medical condition that you have.

5 *Gout*. The Cambridge Diet sole source causes a very slight increase in uric acid during the first two weeks. For the majority of people, this is of no consequence. However, if you suffer from gout and are taking medication, such as Allopurinol, it is important that you should continue the medication while on the diet.

6 *Chronic infections*. The Cambridge Diet can also be beneficial in infectious conditions since it contains all the vitamins, minerals and trace elements which your body needs to fight disease. However, if you are very unwell and are taking a course of antibiotics, it would be advisable not to take the Cambridge Diet sole source until you are better. Remember that it can be used as a nutritional supplement to other food, and you could benefit from using it that way.

7 *Hypoglycemia*. It has been found that people with hypoglycemia often do not have attacks while on the Cambridge Diet. Hypoglycemia is caused by a severe drop in blood glucose about two hours after a meal, particularly one containing a lot of sugar. Since the carbohydrate in the Cambridge Diet is chiefly lactose, which is absorbed very slowly, then hypoglycemia tends not to occur. If it does, than taking six 'half portions' instead of three meals per day seems to help.

8 *Kidney disease*. With certain types of kidney disease, it is important to restrict the amount of protein and electrolytes, such as sodium, that you consume. The Cambridge Diet contains 33g/day of protein and 1.5g/day of sodium (67 mequiv.). Your doctor will use this information in reaching his decision.

Prolonged Sole Source

If you are massively overweight and have a lot to lose, discuss with your doctor the idea of using the Cambridge Diet sole source until you have reached your ideal weight. If he agrees, then you should see him at least every two weeks for a check-up. At the Obesity Clinic at Addenbrooke's Hospital, Cambridge, patients are treated for many months without a break on sole source nutrition. Many patients find that to have a break after four weeks makes life very difficult for them. Once you are on the diet sole source it is very easy to continue, but constant breaks, in which you regain your hunger, can be very disconcerting. The consensus of opinion among doctors is that prolonged use of the Diet sole source should be under strict medical supervision, and I agree.

Obtaining the Product

As explained earlier, the Cambridge Diet is not obtained at retail stores such as supermarkets or chemists. It is sold by people called Cambridge Counsellors, who have taken the diet successfully themselves and want to share their success with others. If you do not know a Cambridge Counsellor but would like to be put in touch with one, write to:

> CAMBRIDGE NUTRITION LIMITED,
> 69-75 THORPE ROAD,
> NORWICH,
> NORFOLK NR1 1HY

Starting the Diet

Before you start the diet, try to work out how long you will have to use the diet sole source before you achieve any real benefit. You should count on about 3½-4 lbs (1.5-1.8 kg) per week. If you have to lose about one stone (6 kg) you will need to be on the diet sole source for at least one month. Therefore plan a period when you do not have many social celebrations, such as your birthday, Christmas or an anniversary. If you are one of those people who have a continual round of social engagements in which you are expected to participate, then you might consider using your holiday for dieting.

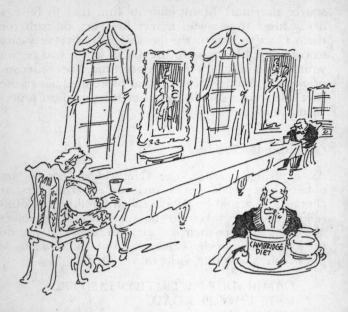

The Great Day

Having chosen the day, look forward to it with pleasure. Tell yourself you are not going to feel hungry (if you do this you will not succumb to eating). If you live on your own, see that the house contains no food whatsoever. If you live with a family then keep the food out of sight and if you usually do the cooking, ask another member of the household to prepare the meals for the first day or two. Remember, you take the Cambridge Diet three times daily in place of regular meals – and *no other food*! Drink plenty of water (I recommend at least eight glasses per day), tea with lemon and black coffee. Also low calorie soda is allowed. Milk in tea and coffee, alcoholic beverages, pure fruit juices and any drink containing sugar or calories are strictly forbidden.

The first three days on your diet will be very exciting, as you lose a great deal of weight every day. It is extremely exhilarating and highly motivating to continue. You will feel better and healthier than you have ever felt in your life because your body is receiving everything it needs.

You will probably feel hungry during the first three days, particularly during the evening. Either do something to keep your mind very occupied or go to bed early with a good book (or partner!). After a few days you will not feel hungry at all. Remember that if you do eat you will feel very hungry, because any extra food will stimulate your appetite. Make a commitment to lose weight and be determined!

Continuing

A few days after starting, you will suddenly realize that you are not hungry at all. In fact, you feel wonderful. Family and friends will comment on how happy you seem to be. You are in a state of euphoria! As long as you remain on the diet you will not be hungry and you will feel happy! If you are a housewife, then you will be able to prepare the family's food and serve them. If, while doing so, you experience a psychological desire for food, then have your Cambridge Diet meal.

Because losing weight can be frustrating, especially during the first three days, the Cambridge Counsellor can be a great help to you and may make the difference between success and failure. If you have any problems or want advice, it is part of his or her job to help you.

You can indulge in all normal activities but you should not be unusually strenuous. Sometimes you will feel a little tired; if you do, then sit down and take a rest.

You should weigh yourself every day at the same time, usually in the morning. You will be delighted with your progress and be very excited with it. This is the real motivation that makes you want to continue. As time goes on, and particularly at the end of the second week, you may experience several days when you do not lose weight. Do not become discouraged. This is a process known as *plateauing*. You are losing fat but retaining water. During this time you may be losing girth faster than weight. For this reason you may find it helpful to use a tape measure in addition to scales. At this stage it is important for you to have faith in the diet. Because, if you continue adhering to the diet, suddenly the weight loss will begin once again as you lose the water you have been retaining.

As already mentioned, the Cambridge Diet is available in a number of different flavours and products. It is helpful to have different flavours throughout the day. In this way you will avoid the monotony which other diets have. On the whole, most people like the flavours and are happy with them. However, if you want to spice them up a bit, it is possible to use your own personal touch by adding calorie-free extracts. Chapter 4 gives recipes for you to try.

Exercise

After you have been on the Cambridge Diet for about five days, and your body has adjusted, consider the idea of indulging in some exercise. This can be very beneficial to your progress and tone up your new body. Chapter 6 gives some suggestions.

Side Effects

Usually there are no side effects, but a few people do experience some minor problems, especially during the first three days. Most of them are common to all diets.

44

The following are some possible causes and the short-term remedies for such side effects:

1 *Headaches* may occur as a result of carbohydrates or caffeine withdrawal. A simple type of headache tablet, e.g. aspirin, taken for a day or two should help the problem.

2 *Constipation.* Since the diet contains only a small amount of bulk you will find that bowel movements are less frequent. However, if you are suffering discomfort due to constipation, then a natural laxative, such as Fybogel (available from chemists) may be taken according to instructions.

3 *Nausea and diarrhoea* may occur as a result of not drinking enough water. The Cambridge Diet contains concentrated minerals and vitamins which may make you feel sick if they are not diluted with water. Drink plenty of liquid after consuming the Cambridge Diet. For instance, you should always have a glass of water or a cup of black tea or coffee or low calorie drink immediately afterwards. In addition to the liquid in which your diet is made up, you should also drink at least three pints (1.75 l) a day.

If the problem persists you may be intolerant to lactose (which is the chief sugar of milk). Perhaps you are one of the unlucky people who cannot digest this sugar, and as a result experience nausea and diarrhoea whenever you drink milk. If you think that this is the case you can predigest the lactose in the Cambridge Diet by using the enzyme lactase. This is sold under the proprietary name Lactaid, and is available through your local chemist. Just add four drops to your reconstituted diet, stir, refrigerate for 24 hours and drink. However, during the process quite a lot of vitamin C may be destroyed. You should, therefore, supplement the diet with at least

45

100 mg per day of vitamin C. (Tablets are available from your local chemist.)

4 *Dizziness* is most often caused by the diuretic effect of the diet. Drink plenty of water and you will find that it will usually disappear. For those who are prone to attacks of faintness, it is important to avoid what is called 'postural hypertension'. This occurs when one rises from a chair too rapidly and feels faint and dizzy. In such circumstances, remember not to rush up quickly from your sitting position but to take life a little more slowly!

5 *Mouth odour*. After you have been on the diet sole source for a few days your family and friends may tell you that your breath smells. Explain that this is quite natural and ask them to bear with it. The reason why it happens is that since you have stopped eating your mouth is not being completely cleaned by the food you chew. A partial solution is to brush your teeth often and to use a mouthwash frequently. There is also available low calorie chewing gum (not ordinary gum) which will achieve the cleansing effect of food.

6 *Fatigue*. Some people who lead a very strenuous life and are used to a job which is physically demanding, or alternatively play vigorous games, find that they are more fatigued than usual. The solution here is to take life a bit easier, perhaps give up sport for a week or two and go to bed earlier. On the other hand, many people who are not used to a strenuous life find that they have a good deal more energy and can achieve much more physically than they did before going on the diet.

7 *Irritability*. Most people feel very happy whilst taking the Cambridge Diet, but occasionally there are those

who feel slightly irritable. This is usually at the beginning of the diet and with time the effect wears off and one's mood changes for the better.

8 *Persistent side effects*. The advantage of losing weight should certainly override any short-term discomfort you may experience. However, should the side effects continue it is important to consult your Cambridge Counsellor or doctor for further advice.

Add a Meal Interval

If you are not under constant medical supervision you should use the Cambridge Diet sole source for no more than four weeks. You must then add one 400 calorie meal to your three daily helpings of Cambridge Diet for seven days and Chapter 17 gives typical menu examples. If you are lucky you will probably lose a little weight during the break period. If you have not reached your ideal body weight, go back to using the Cambridge Diet sole source after your week's break.

Cambridge Slim Meals

If, by the end of the fourth week of taking the Cambridge Diet sole source, target weight is not achieved, a 400 calorie meal must be added to the three servings of the diet for one week. During this fifth week weight loss will still take place.

As the preparation and cooking of a 400 calorie meal can be time consuming as well as inexact, Cambridge Nutrition Limited has developed a range of meals, with one of the UK's leading suppliers of groceries. When cooked with rice or pasta, each meal provides the necessary 400 calories needed during the crucial fifth week whilst on the diet.

There are four varieties to choose from, Chicken Curry, Beef Curry, Chilli con Carne and Bolognaise Sauce with Minced Beef. The meat used in these products has been devised so that they have a very low fat content. On average the amount of fat is less than 2% of the product's weight when reconstituted with water.

Cambridge Slim Desserts

Even commited slimmers love to indulge in desserts and after numerous requests from successful Cambridge Diet slimmers, a range of 50 calorie desserts was launched.

These products are designed for use during the fifth week of The Cambridge Diet regime and during the weight maintenance when target weight has been achieved and eating habits adjusted.

In three varieties, Chocolate, Strawberry and Banana, the desserts are pleasant to eat and offer good value for money.

Weight Maintenance Programme

When you have reached your ideal weight you really will feel healthier and fitter than you have done for many years. I am sure you will want to continue to feel this way, to maintain your weight and retain your new slim figure. This is when you embark on the Cambridge Plan Weight Maintenance Programme. The next chapter explains how to keep the weight off.

CHAPTER FOUR

KEEPING THE WEIGHT OFF

Using the Cambridge Diet, you may, for the first time, have been able to lose a lot of weight. That was the easy part; keeping the weight off is more difficult. However, the availability of the Cambridge Diet makes the task simpler. At our clinic in Cambridge, we have records now of scores of people who have reduced their weight by 50 to 100 lbs (22-45 kg) and have still kept their weight off over the course of many years. How did they do it?

The key of success is to use the Cambridge Diet three times a day as a nutritional supplement, even when you are eating ordinary food. When your body is supplied with complete nutrition, your appetite is more easily satisfied and you do not crave excessive quantities of food.

Then it is important to keep a regular check on your weight – if possible every day. When your body weight is increased by more than five pounds above your ideal weight, it is time to take prompt action. This can be done by cutting out one or two meals each day and continuing with your Cambridge Diet meal. Alternatively, you may find it easier to go on the diet as sole source for a few days, say Monday and Friday. Very often, I myself find it easier in the working week not to eat so much food but to indulge more at the weekend.

As time goes by, people who have been plagued by being overweight for most of their lives become slim, and attain great confidence. The Cambridge Diet is a very powerful tool with which you can control your weight.

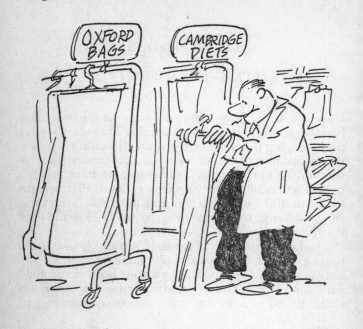

Cutting Down on the Calories

You became overweight because you consumed more calories than your body needed. Thus, to maintain your newly found set-point, you must change your eating habits for ever. The Cambridge Diet, eaten three times daily, will provide 330 calories. This allows you around 1,500 calories for additional food.

You may be one of those extremely clever people who, armed with a calculator, can immediately tot up the calorie content of each meal. If you are like me, you plan your meals according to broad principles and tackle the problem by avoiding foods of high calorie value. In this respect, you will find the following hints helpful:

1 *Avoid fat.* Fat (and oils) contain nine calories per gram, which is two and a quarter times more than protein or carbohydrate. If you are to control your weight, it is extremely important that you restrict the quantities of fat and oils that you eat.

   Avoid fried foods and fatty foods. Wherever possible, grill and poach but rarely fry. (If you do need to fry, use a non-stick pan.) Especially avoid fried chips (French fries), potato crisps and food fried in batter. Eat boiled and poached, rather than fried eggs.

   When vegetables are cooked, do not mix them with butter.

   With salads, use a low-calorie salad dressing, vinegar or lemon juice, herbs and spices.

   Avoid foods made with pastry such as meat and fruit pies, fatty croissants, danish pastries, and sausage rolls.

   Use skimmed milk instead of full cream milk.

   Use low fat yoghurt instead of cream.

   Use low fat cheese (e.g. cottage cheese) and have cream and hard cheese just occasionally.

   Use less butter and margarine on bread.

   Eat nuts occasionally but never more than a two-ounce packet at a time (they are very high in calories).

   Use lean cuts of meat and wherever possible cut the fat off meat and eat only the lean part.

   Eat grilled chicken, without the skin, and white fish more frequently, since these are less fatty.

2 *Restrict alcohol.* Drink only in moderation, since alcohol contains seven calories per gram (one-and-three-quarter times more than carbohydrate or protein). Limit your drinking to no more than one or

two drinks per day. If you drink at lunch time, skip it for dinner.

Mineral water with ice and a slice of lemon makes an excellent drink at parties and is extremely fashionable.

3 *Restrict salt*. Too much salt in the diet can cause high blood pressure and fluid retention.

Avoid, as far as possible, adding salt at the table. If you have to use any at all, substitute one of the new mineral salts (in which part of the salt is replaced by potassium salts).

Most of the salt we eat is put into manufactured (e.g. canned and packaged) foods. Thus use unsalted, rather than salted butter, and also unsalted nuts. Eat little of salty fish (kippers, smoked and canned fish) and potato crisps. When cooking your own cakes and pastries or Yorkshire pudding go easy on the salt and use the special mineral salt referred to above.

4 *Eat fibre*. Fruit and vegetables and wholemeal bread contain a lot of roughage (fibre). Special crispbreads and crisps containing bran are also recommended. Besides filling you up and curbing your appetite, it's healthy.

5 *Restrict sugar*. Although sugar is not as calorific as fat or alcohol, it is still a highly concentrated source of calories, with no other nutritional value. Avoid sugar drinks (cordials, sweet fizzy sodas and Cola). Use one of the low-calorie varieties instead. If you must sweeten coffee or tea use a sugar substitute with one of the calorie-free sweeteners, such as saccharine or the new sweetener, aspartame (Candarel). The latter is excellent, indistinguishable from sugar and leaves no after-taste. Most of the sweeteners are unstable if heated, so if you are sweetening stewed fruit, the sweetener should be added after cooking and not before.

In many manufactured foods, sugar is often combined with fat. Sweets, chocolate and creamy cakes should be treated with suspicion!

Healthy Eating

At this point you will have reached the conclusion that everything you like is strictly taboo and fattening. You may be one of those people who loves fish and chips, cream gateaux and salty hamburgers with French fries. How is it possible to eat sensibly and lead a happy life?

There is a sensible approach, which I adopt myself. Most of the time, about six days a week, I am fairly strict and eat very sensibly, according to the above rules. Then once a week I will throw caution to the winds and indulge. Now and again I will have fish and chips and enjoy it tremendously. The same applies to scones with strawberry jam and cream. Most nutritionists I know do exactly the same.

Recommended Menus

To help you in your search for interesting and tasty food, Chapter 16 provides a number of typical low-calorie menus, some of which are gourmet and others which are more practical. You will find these are a helpful guide to the type of dishes you should be eating as part of your permanent eating plan.

The Secret

The secret of keeping weight off is that the Cambridge Diet is always available whenever you need it. In our original experiments at the West Middlesex Hospital, one lady originally weighing 320 lbs (145 kg) lost about

155 lbs (70 kg) in hospital. While there, she was adamant that she would never regain her weight, having spent one year of her life in hospital losing it. But she failed.

Unfortunately, after discharge she moved to another part of the country and it became impossible to contact her. Two years later, she turned up at the hospital having regained all the weight she had lost, and was even heavier.

There were no supplies of Cambridge Diet available for her maintenance programme in those days. If we were dealing with her case today, I believe it would be a different story, as shown by countless others who have followed her, but have succeeded in keeping slim.

A Permanent Change

One of the most severe criticisms of the Cambridge Diet made by some psychologists and hospital dieticians, is that it does not change people's eating habits in the long term and is therefore useless, particularly for maintaining weight loss. To these armchair critics it is just another fad diet. Nothing could be further from the truth as anyone can vouch who has used the diet as a sole source of nutrition for several weeks. For the first time one realizes that vast quantities of food are not indispensable to life. It trains you to live without having food continually on your mind and the experience has a beneficial effect on most people. There is ample proof that the Cambridge maintenance plan does achieve excellent results.

The Statistics

A survey was made recently by The Opinion Research Corporation of San Francisco, California, of about 500 people who had lost more than 50 lbs (22 kg) in body weight and continued using the Cambridge Diet for at least one year afterwards. During that year, 30 per cent had continued to lose weight, 30 per cent had kept their weight stationary and the remaining 40 per cent increased their body weight. However, of this latter group, the increase in weight had only been a mean of 20 lbs (9 kg), so that almost everyone had still lost weight. Overall, if one looks at the results of other diets which have been studied in a similar way, they are abysmal. They report that 95 per cent of all people who lose weight regain it again three years later.

Attaining a new set point at a lower body weight is now possible for everyone, including yourself.

The Achievement

For some people it is still a struggle and I end this chapter with a story which illustrates how one person was able to succeed, despite the severe handicap of requiring only 600 calories per day. Her name is Betty Stevens and here is her story.

Personal Story of Betty Stevens, St Albans, Herts

'Even as a young child I was overweight. As a little girl I had rheumatic fever and from that point I steadily began to gain weight. I went on all sorts of diets and I would go down a bit but then it would start going up and up again. Mostly I was on calorie controlled diets of 800 to 1,000 calories. On the 1,000 calorie diet I would begin to put weight on again.

'I have had to be on diets all my life. My mother was overweight and my older brother still has problems. He always says we couldn't even raise a glass of water without putting on weight!

'I had been under the St Albans Hospital Clinic at various times and had been treated by the dietician there for about five years. During this time I was up and down, but then during the last year I began going up and up again – even on an 800 calorie diet. I became so depressed and discouraged at gaining weight on 800 calories that the dietician finally said that there just was no other diet that she could give me and suggested that I go back to my doctor. He tested me for everything he could, including my thyroid gland, but just couldn't find anything wrong. He finally said he would try to get me into the Obesity Clinic at Addenbrooke's Hospital, Cambridge – it was the only thing left for me to do.

'In July 1983 I went to the clinic at Addenbrooke's and I weighed 15 stone (210 lbs; 95 kg). In six months' time I was down to a weight of 9st. 8 lbs (132 lbs; 60 kg), a loss of 78 lbs (35 kg).

'I felt wonderful all the time on the diet. My father says I was full of life! I never felt tired and had far more energy than on any of the other diets I'd been on. My depression was gone and I had a feeling of happiness the whole time. I stayed sole source for the entire six months (even at Christmas time, I never had a bite to eat). I was determined to get down.

'It was fantastic. I wasn't very hungry and felt satisfied all the time, even at the beginning. I cooked meals for my father the whole time I was dieting. I find that cooking relaxes me. I really love cooking, of any sort, and after I'd come home from work I'd make cakes and pastries. It just never bothered me. I wasn't hungry.

'The weight had been getting me down and after having been so depressed and desperate I was quite happy with my instant results and was determined to stay with it.

'When I started the diet I was wearing a size 22 and now can get into a 12. People pass me on the street or see me at work and don't even recognize me.

'I am a secretary, and all of my bosses and the men at

56

my office were so encouraging to me – they were fantastic at helping me. They tell me they have noticed a tremendous difference in me mentally (I'm sharper and brighter) as well as being physically more active. As I got rid of the weight I became more enthusiastic about everything at work. I had more confidence in myself, I looked better and felt better. Now I could buy clothes that were stylish. I hadn't been able to get anything nice in my size before (they don't make stylish clothes in those sizes)!

'When I began weight maintenance I tried taking the Cambridge Diet and adding two meals a day but I began putting on a bit (just too much for my liking) so I learned that to maintain my weight I would need to continue taking the Cambridge Diet three times a day and just have one small meal. I must hold to about 600 calories a day. In fact I have lost even a bit more weight on maintenance – and now weigh about 9st. 3lbs (129 lbs; 58.5 kg).

'Whenever I see I might be putting on more weight I just go sole source for two or three days and take it right off again. Mostly I maintain very well at 600 calories and have it under control for the first time in my life.

'My skin isn't flabby and I don't look pale, thin or haggard as I did on other diets. My skin, hair and nails look so healthy. In fact everybody says I look fantastic! I never feel a bit lethargic or tired. It's just been wonderful.

'If I go out anywhere I take the Cambridge Diet along with me. While everyone else is eating sandwiches or having coffee I have my Cambridge Diet. As I am a District Cub Scout Leader I have 29 packs and must visit the scout camps. They used always to try to get me to stop and have a meal, but they're used to me now. I even cooked at two camps this year, but I have my Cambridge Diet and do just fine – it's easy for me.

'I have found a new and happy life now and I honestly wouldn't want to be without the Cambridge Diet – ever!'

CHAPTER FIVE

FOR NUTRITION

There is more to a healthy life than just being thin. Many of the diseases which affect our lives are due to faulty nutrition. Among them are coronary heart disease, high blood pressure, stroke and cancer. All these diseases occur in thin as well as fat people. Also, nutritional surveys have shown that many people do not consume the recommended level of many vitamins, minerals and trace elements. It is common for obese people to comment that after weight reduction they feel fitter and healthier than they have ever done in their life. They continue to take the Cambridge Diet, not only for weight maintenance but as a nutritional supplement, as it contains all the recommended daily allowances of the above nutrients.

Even naturally thin people take the Cambridge Diet three times a day just for nutrition. By doing so, they help to prevent diseases occurring and also ensure that they are not deficient in nutrients.

There are a number of very good reasons why the Cambridge Diet is potentially beneficial in prolonging life and it fits in well with modern concepts of the perfect nutritional life-style. I shall therefore discuss these concepts in more detail.

Coronary Heart Disease

There is still much controversy on this subject in the scientific and medical world and it is not surprising that the public is often very confused. Briefly, animal fats including dairy products and meat fats, etc., raise the level of a substance in the blood called cholesterol. It is this substance which accumulates in the inner walls of arteries, notably in the coronary arteries. Those people who are susceptible to attacks of coronary thrombosis often, but not always, have a high level of blood cholesterol. Vegetable oils, like corn, sunflower seed and safflower oil are thought to lower the level of blood cholesterol. For this reason, many nutritionists recommend that these replace animal fats. Vegetable oils are rich in what are called poly-unsaturated fatty acids and the animal fats are rich in saturated fats.

In industrialized countries, the total consumption of fat is about 40 per cent of all the calories eaten. Public health authorities are now recommending that it should be cut as low as 30 per cent, and some authorities suggest even lower levels. The PS ratio of the fat consumed should be increased. That means that the proportion of poly-unsaturated (present in vegetable oils) to saturated fatty acids (present in animal fats) should be increased.

The Cambridge Diet contains no animal fats whatsoever. In fact, it is very low in fat and contains only 3 grams per day, of which two-thirds is poly-unsaturated. If one were recommending a diet which would be suitable as a prevention for coronary heart disease, the Cambridge Diet would take top place. It contributes virtually no fats to the total intake and when eaten with other low fat foods would be instrumental in cutting down the total fat calories to those which are recommended.

The Cambridge Diet is also cholesterol free. And, although many people believe that dietary cholesterol is not important, some nutritionists recommend that foods rich in cholesterol should be avoided.

The cause of coronary heart disease is unknown and although the saturated/poly-unsaturated fat theory is widely held, it cannot explain many of the deaths which occur from this prevalent disease. There are speculations about the effect of other nutrients. One scientist, Leslie Klevay of North Dakota, believes that a deficiency of copper or a low ratio of copper to zinc in the diet may be important. There is much to support his view. In a recent survey in The Netherlands, it was found that the tissues of people dying with extensive atherosclerosis of the coronary arteries had a lower copper content than people with smaller amounts of disease. As atherosclerosis in the coronaries is a major contributory factor towards coronary heart disease, an increased intake of copper might prevent it.

The intake of copper in Westernized populations is rather low and well below the 2 milligrams per day which is recommended by nutritionists. The Cambridge Diet contains the recommended daily allowance. Should it be true that lack of copper is a contributory factor towards coronary heart disease, the inclusion of the Cambridge Diet three times a day would be an important preventive measure.

Another group of nutritionists believes that our diet should contain more fibre, that is, the fibrous material present in whole-grain flour, fruit and vegetables. They suggest that a deficiency of this important nutrient might also contribute to coronary heart disease. The Cambridge Diet does not contain a great deal of fibre – only about three grams per day. Attempts are being made to increase the fibre content of the Cambridge Diet at this time. However, for people on a maintenance regime, it is certainly recommended that they eat as much fibre as they can. I would suggest that whenever possible they should eat wholewheat products and plenty of fresh fruit and vegetables.

High Blood Pressure

The incidence of high blood pressure in the population is increasing, because people are living longer and blood pressure increases with age. High blood pressure causes damage in two ways; either by precipitating coronary heart disease or by causing stroke. Thus a control of your blood pressure is extremely important if these two diseases are to be prevented. At a recent conference on diet and high blood pressure, in Finland, the experts decided that the main nutritional factors which could contribute are:

1 Too much salt in the diet
2 Not enough potassium
3 Too little poly-unsaturated fats
4 Excessive alcohol intake

Much of our knowledge of these factors comes from population studies. For instance, some Japanese eat vast quantities of salt daily, because it is used in the preservation of the fish they eat. They can consume as much as 20 to 35 grams of salt per day. Their most prevalent cause of death is stroke, caused by very high blood pressure.

It has been suggested that the epidemic of high blood pressure in industrialized countries could be prevented if the salt content could be reduced drastically. Health authorities recommend that the current intake of about 12 grams per day should be reduced to one-third, about four grams per day. It is interesting that potassium salts counteract this effect of salt and there is a move towards increasing its intake.

The Cambridge Diet makes an important contribution in this area. It contains only 1.5 grams of sodium per day but is very high in potassium (2 grams per day). This means that it is a moderately low sodium, high potassium diet. Although it does contain some poly-unsaturated fatty acids, which are also beneficial towards lowering blood pressure, these are in rather small amounts. Therefore, it is important to supplement the Cambridge Diet with vegetable oils – for example corn oil – when on the maintenance programme.

It is only a high intake of alcohol which increases blood pressure, and one or two drinks a day have no effect whatever. Thus, if you think it is important to drink alcohol, you should not exceed this quantity, otherwise you may be increasing your blood pressure.

Cancer

Our knowledge of the importance of nutrition in the prevention of cancer has increased remarkably during the last few years. The nutrients which appear to be involved are; dietary fat, fibre, vitamins A, C and E, and also selenium. A high level of fat in the diet seems to be related to a higher incidence of cancer in animals. In this respect, vegetable oils are no different and may be even worse than animal fats. For this reason, many health authorities recommend that the total fat consumption should be reduced and there should be no net increase in vegetable oils. Therefore, a decrease in total fat levels could be of great value in the prevention of two major diseases which affect us; coronary heart disease and cancer.

In experimental studies in animals, it is found that vitamin E and selenium can stop the formation of chemical substances known as 'free radicals', because they are antioxidants (prevent oxidation). There is one important theory which states that free radicals are one of the major promoters of cancer in the body and any measure which cuts down their formation is worthwhile. The Cambridge Diet provides ample vitamin E and selenium. Also, in animals, vitamin A has been found to be very effective in preventing cancers caused by the introduction of cancer-forming substances. The vitamin apparently works by affecting the surfaces of cells so that they are less susceptible to other substances which may cause cancer.

Vitamin C works in a different way. Many foodstuffs contain nitrites as preservatives. When nitrites enter the stomach they are converted into cancer-forming substances called nitrosamines. Vitamin C prevents the formation of these nitrosamines and has been shown to be very effective experimentally in animals.

To summarize, the high vitamin A, C, E and selenium content of the Cambridge Diet is potentially very useful if it is indeed the case that vitamins and minerals prevent cancer.

Dietary fibre is also thought by some experts to prevent colon cancer. For this reason maybe it is important to include fibre in a maintenance diet, as suggested above.

Longevity

Although many people are now living to a greater age, the natural life span, that is the maximum time people live, is still no more than it was 100 or even 1,000 years ago. Most people die in their seventies or eighties, and although more people now reach that age, the total life span is not increasing.

During the last century, people died young from the infectious diseases, such as tuberculosis, pneumonia and cholera, which were rife within the population because of poor public health standards. With the greater awareness of the causes of these diseases and the introduction of antibiotics, very few people now die from them. However, as more people live longer, they die from diseases of old age, or more particularly from coronary heart disease, cancer and stroke.

A major question for the future is whether it will be possible to increase the life span to 100 or 120 years or even more. One physician, Dr J. Walford of UCLA, believes it may be possible to do this. He expresses his view in a book, *Maximum Life Span*. The method he suggests is to eat less – much less. His theory is based on work on experimental animals. For instance, rats which are fed on about 50 per cent of what they normally eat, increase their life span up to 60 per cent, providing that the diet still contains adequate vitamins, minerals and other important nutrients. In other words, the secret of longevity is 'under-nutrition' without malnutrition. Other scientists have shown that intermittent fasting (that is, cutting out food for a few days) also has an effect on increasing life span in rats. Animals fed a high quality diet, as much as they wanted, but made to fast completely every second day, lived over 1,000 days compared with only 800 days for those which had normal rations.

How can a decreased intake of foods increase your life span? The answer may lie in your body temperature. Animals kept in a cool temperature live much longer than those who are warm. This happens when you go without food. Your body temperature decreases and your metabolism is slowed down. These are the two factors which are thought to increase life span.

Dr Walford recommends a total abstinence from food for two successive days every week and a healthy moderate diet during the other five days. When not eating food, it is important to take other non-calorific nutrients, such as vitamins, minerals and trace elements. If one were looking for a diet which would fit in with his concept, it would be the Cambridge Diet. There are many people who are taking it not only twice a week sole source, but very often five days or more. If Dr Walford is right, then people who carry out this regime over many years should live a great deal longer. Time will tell if he is right!

The Cambridge Diet as a Nutritional Supplement

There are many of us who believe that the most important contribution the Cambridge Diet can make in our
civilization is to provide good, basic nutrition. Three
Cambridge meals every day will provide all the recommended daily allowances of the vitamins, minerals and
trace elements. There is no other single food of 330
calories per day which achieves this end. It has an
enormous potential in preventing malnutrition, particularly in children, pregnant and nursing women and
the elderly.

Because the Cambridge Diet is very palatable, it is
well received by elderly people who very often have
problems in chewing food or who become uninterested
or too infirm to prepare good, nourishing food.
Toddlers often reach a stage of being unconcerned
about food and will go for a long time ignoring what is
put in front of them. But it has been reported by many
counsellors that a child will always want a drink of what
he sees his mother drinking. The many varieties of
flavours appeal to a child and while he is getting what he
thinks is a special grown-up drink, he is in fact, getting
all the nutrition he needs.

Athletes

It was not long after its introduction in the United
States that professional athletes and team players found
out the great value of the Cambridge Diet as a nutritional supplement. Among the first to use it were
members of the Philadelphia Eagles football team,
whose coach, Otto Davis, insisted that all his players
should use it regularly as part of their normal training.
Some of the benefits claimed were a more sustained
energy level during the game and an increased speed of
healing of injuries. The early success of the Philadel-

phia Eagles was so remarkable that many other football teams copied them. For quite a time the Eagles had an advantage and were winning most of their games. Eventually, all the other teams, having 'got the message', took the Cambridge Diet and the Eagles lost their advantage.

There is another way in which the Cambridge Diet can help sportsmen and women, and that is when they retire. Dennis Franks, a former centre for the Philadel-

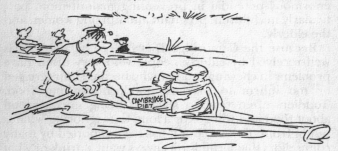

phia Eagles, weighed about 19 stone (270 lbs; 122 kg), much of which was healthy muscle and important to him as a football player. After retiring from the game, he started the Cambridge Diet and lost 14 lbs (6.35 kg) in 3 days and 42 lbs (19 kg) in 3 weeks. He runs an average of 2 miles (1.6 km) and does 1 hour of weight lifting per day. Many heavy-weight sportsmen die young because after they retire their muscles turn to fat and they do not decrease their body weight to the ideal. It is very important that they should decrease their weight and many of them have found that the use of the Cambridge Diet is a speedy and effective way to do it.

In the United States, large numbers of people now regularly use the Cambridge Diet for nutrition, and the same is beginning to happen in Britain. These people believe it is beneficial, because they feel better, have a higher energy level and have a firm belief that a good nutritional basis can lead to a healthier and longer life.

According to all good nutritional principles, they should be right! They should develop fewer of the diseases of Western-style civilization such as coronary heart disease, cancer and strokes; and because of their lowered metabolism, they should live longer. It is an interesting and important human experiment – and we shall know the answer only in twenty or thirty years from now. I am firmly convinced that they will be proved right.

Case History

As an example of how people find the Cambridge Diet of great benefit for nutrition, I give the story of Eleanor Harnish, who has multiple sclerosis. Although the Cambridge Diet did not cure her disease, it greatly improved the quality of her life.

Personal Story of Eleanor Harnish, Cambridge (formerly of Norman, Oklahoma)

'In January of 1972 I was diagnosed as having multiple sclerosis. This ended ten years of physical and mental anguish in trying to discover what my "health problems" could be. At one time or another I have suffered most of the typical MS symptoms; blurred vision, disorientation, incontinence, headaches, leg spasms, numbness, poor memory and loss of concentration, shuffling walk, lack of coordination and the worst problem of all, severe fatigue attacks. Twice it was necessary to spend some time in a wheelchair and on fore-arm crutches or a cane. I have had many years of ups and downs in learning to cope with the unpredictable days of an MS way of life.

'In mid-April of 1981, while living in the USA, my husband and I were introduced to the Cambridge Diet by very close friends. I was very concerned about being able to take the diet as a sole source of nutrition with this illness, as I felt that going without food would cause me to become too weak and fatigued. However, with encouragement from my doctor and from our Cambridge Counsellor, I decided to give it a try.

'As both my husband and I were overweight, we were delighted with our successful and quick weight loss: 30 lbs (13 kg) for my husband and 35 lbs (16 kg) for me. You can imagine my great surprise to have found a wonderful side-effect (besides the benefit of losing weight)! I began to have more energy. Lots of it! For an MS patient this is a fantastic blessing.

'I would like to tell you some other interesting observations that we began to notice during the years I have been on the Cambridge Diet. In May of 1982 I developed a sinus infection which quickly brought on another problem, laryngitis. Within a week I had developed bronchitis. I was over-tired and under stress (both devastating problems for an MS victim). It was impossible for the doctor to prescribe medication as I am allergic to so many antibiotics and many medications beneficial in treating an infection. Whenever I had become this ill with infections in the past, it had always brought on an MS attack. I was worried! With my doctor's approval I put myself to bed, and took Cambridge sole source for a week. To my great joy I was up and feeling great in less than two weeks. I not only had beaten the infection but the best news of all – no MS attack!

'For some reason I find that going sole source when I am having an MS attack (in addition to some rest) seems to be of great benefit to me. Before Cambridge came into my life I had never been able to throw off an MS attack once it was in progress.

'In reviewing my past medical records I find that from January 1972 to 1980 I had been hospitalized with varying symptoms of MS problems from one to three times a year. Each hospital admission was for an average of around three weeks. I can only say that I am terriby thrilled to have stayed out of hospital during the past 5 years – of which I have been on Cambridge for 4½ years. If I could only convey to you what this has meant, not only to me but to the lives of my husband and family!

'During these past 4½ years I have felt great and have had marvelous days without my usual afternoons and evenings of fatigue. I still can't get over having energy again and being able to live a fairly normal life. There has been a decrease in urinary problems, I am walking better and the numbness problems have greatly improved. My powers of concentration are better and I am doing some rather remarkable and interesting things. The greatest blessing for me has been the lack of trips to the hospital!

'Of course I still have MS. And occasionally I have some minor symptoms, but I seem to be able to throw off most problems quickly and have suffered no serious attacks. I do watch my stress level and try not to tire myself and I always take my Cambridge formula three times a day. I do find that the longer I am on Cambridge the better my health becomes.

'I haven't reached this point overnight, and I encourage anyone with either multiple sclerosis or any other serious illness to just remain faithful to the nutritional programme of taking Cambridge three times daily. It takes time for the body to try and heal itself!

'In no way do I make claim that the Cambridge formula is a cure for multiple sclerosis or any other disease. I can honestly say, however, that I have never felt so well in 20 years. I am convinced that getting my body into metabolic balance and feeding it with proper vitamins, minerals, trace elements and nutrients has certainly made a tremendous difference in my symptoms. It has helped my body throw off infection and serious MS attacks. I also must add that I am convinced that using Cambridge for nutritional value is just common sense. It's good preventive medicine!'

CHAPTER SIX

EXERCISE

Very few people can lose weight just by exercise alone. To quote an experiment done in Sweden, Dr Krotkiewski, one of that country's leading experts, saw sixteen patients who were consuming the Cambridge Diet, and divided them into two groups. One group had a strenuous work-out in the gym three times a week, and the other group just sat down and watched. At the end of three weeks he found there was no difference in weight-loss, even though the exercise group expended 1,650 more calories in physical activity.

To burn up 1 lb (450g) of body fat you need to expend about 3,500 calories so the maximum effect would theoretically be only ½ lb (225 g), an amount too small to measure in small groups of people who individually have a wide variation in weight losses.

This is not to say that I do not feel exercise is important. On the contrary, it is absolutely essential for long term weight maintenance and anyone trying to keep physically fit. Besides slowing down the ageing process, exercise is thought by many doctors to reduce the risk of coronary heart disease.

But there are great dangers in someone undertaking strenuous exercise when they are unused to it. If you are seriously interested, then it is mandatory to consult your doctor, especially if you are over the age of forty. He will check that you have no underlying medical condition which contra-indicates your starting. Quite a few people have ended up with a coronary attack after strenous exercise because they were unaware that they had coronary heart disease.

The Cambridge Diet provides a means of losing weight rapidly and dramatically. Since overweight people are usually not very keen on exercise and lose weight easily on the diet, they tend to give exercise no

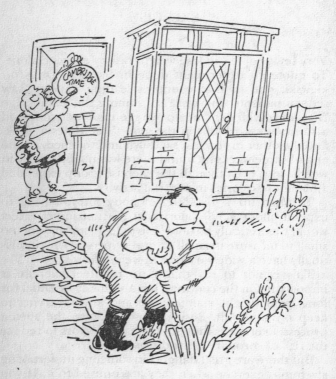

further thought. This is a pity because in the long term exercise should be of supreme importance in weight maintenance. The reason for this is that exercise can increase the ratio of muscle to fat in the body. Muscle tissue requires much more energy than fat for maintenance and a person's normal resting metabolism is largely dependent on how much muscle is present in the body. When you exercise, your muscles increase in size and you will continually burn up more energy even when you are not exercising but just sitting still.

Whilst you are taking the Cambridge Diet as the sole source of nutrition, it is unlikely that you will build up much muscle, as the number of calories are very restricted. However, on the maintenance plan, when you supplement the diet with additional calories and much more protein, the ratio of muscle to fat will automatically increase, providing you exercise as well.

In today's fast-paced, quick-moving world many of us find that the greatest amount of exercise we get is what we expend walking from our dwellings to our cars or the bus. Of course, we do occasionally take the dog for a walk or spend a day or two swimming while on holiday, but for the most part, we have become much less active than our ancestors, while in fact, eating a great deal more.

If you are very overweight, or have been quite inactive and happen to be over forty, your feelings about exercise might parallel those of a well-known comedienne who said, 'The first time I see a jogger smiling, I'll consider trying it,' or another who commented, 'My idea of exercise is a good, brisk sit.' If you have similar feelings, let me encourage you to start exercising; but I suggest you wait until you have been on the Cambridge Diet at least four to five days and then continue even when you reach your ideal body weight, because it is then that you will reap maximum benefit. You should then achieve a new set-point, that is, a new weight level around which your weight oscillates.

In my opinion 'aerobics' are the best exercises, and for those who are unaware of what aerobics are, I will attempt an explanation. Our knowledge of the benefits of exercise has taken a huge leap forward in recent years. It is now recognized that of the many different types of exercises, the results you can obtain are quite different. Exercises can be divided into two types: aerobic and anaerobic. The word aerobic literally means *with* air, whilst anaerobic means *without* air. When exercise is aerobic, large quantities of oxygen are consumed by the muscles and fat, instead of carbohydrate being burned. Thus, aerobics are a great advantage to someone who wants to lose weight, because the body fat is burned in preference to other energy stores. Moreover, body metabolism is speeded up for many hours after a brisk work-out.

What exercises are aerobic? Any strenuous, continuous use of your muscles for at least 12 minutes. Thus, swimming, cycling, jogging, walking (for 45 minutes), cross-country skiing, roller and ice skating are all aerobic, providing they are continuous. Other stop-go sports such as tennis, weight-lifting, football, golf and other team sports are not aerobic but anaerobic.

What are the further benefits of aerobics? It can do wonders for your heart and lungs and general body metabolism. It produces changes in your brain chemistry which are, in many ways, similar to the benefits of sleeping pills, drugs which lower blood pressure, tranquillisers, anti-depressants, without the side-effects one normally gets when taking these types of drugs.

I recommend that you practise aerobic exercises at least three times per week (remembering that the critical time for their performance is at least 12 minutes). In the course of time your heart and lungs will benefit by becoming stronger, they will be able to handle more easily a sudden demand for energy without being overworked. The heart rests longer between beats and this is reflected by a drop in pulse rate.

In Chapter 17, exercise is discussed in more detail. Among the different types of exercise considered are swimming, jogging and running, gym exercises and weight lifting, aerobic dancing, cycling, and walking. If you want to keep fit as well as slim you are advised to read it.

I now present the heartening story of a fat man who achieved his ambition to run in the Cambridge marathon.

Personal Story of Anthony Crouch, Cambridge

'Twenty months ago I always had an answer for being fat – "I've always been fat," or "I'm big boned and very muscular." You see, I had picked up weight from the day I was born. I've always had weight problems. As a child I was called Fatty Arbuckle. This always hurt, but you have to put on a strong face and be a broad-shouldered person. I've been up to as much as 22 stone (308 lbs; 140 kg) when I was about 24 years old.

'Oh, the diets I've tried – it's unbelievable. I've tried this and that, been in hospital and on special diets. Nothing worked.

'For years I had suffered severe pains in my back which went right down into my right leg. I had seen an osteopath because I thought I had a bad nerve problem but nothing ever came out of it, so I went to the doctor and he suggested that I lose a bit of weight and he gave me some pills which could be addictive (amphetamines). They gave me a feeling of being really up and all tensed. They worked for a short while but gave no great loss of weight. Then the doctor said I really needed to reduce the intake of food. This went on for years and years.

'The pains were getting so bad I had to have up to eight pain killers a day for the pain and on a cold and wet day I was in absolute agony.

'Eventually, my doctor said he would book me into Addenbrooke's Hospital to see someone. I thought I was going to see someone about my pain, but when I arrived they weighed me in and as I looked around I said to myself, "There are a lot of people here who are overweight", and then I suddenly realized what I was attending hospital for.

'And so, I went on the Cambridge Diet for five days and when I went back to hospital and found that in actual fact I had lost in the region of 10 lbs (4.5 kg), I was amazed. This was the first weight I'd lost that quickly in years.

'Gradually over the weeks, I started to lose quite large amounts of weight, then levelled off to 3 or 4 lbs (1-2 kg) per week, then to about 2 lbs (1 kg) a week. Eventually I got to my goal of 11½ stones (161 lbs; 73 kg). I lost 80 lbs (36 kg) in 6 months and I've kept it off.

'While I was losing this weight I began feeling a lot fitter. I had completely forgotten about the pains in my legs and back. This past winter, 1983-4, was the first in years without all that pain. Sure, on a few days I had a couple of twinges but nothing like I'd had in past years! And as I was feeling so well I started doing many things I hadn't been able to do. For one, I started jogging. I finally determined that I was going to get all my weight off and do the local Cambridge Sinclair Marathon. Everyone was sceptical and said, "You think you can do that?" Well, I knew I could do it.

'I started in the mornings, going only half a mile and gradually was going long distances without being totally worn out. I had more energy and felt physically fit. Much better than I had in most of my life. I even play squash three times a week now. In fact at work I used to be so tired I'd fall asleep during tea breaks but now they tell me to slow down and take it easy – to stop tearing around!

'The first year that I entered the Marathon, in July 1983, I got a fairly good time, but this year, with all the weight off, I took 4 minutes 38 seconds off of last year's time – and at 40, I'm a year older!

'I was pleased, not so much about my time, but just that I'd completed something I had set out to do (not to win but just to run in the Marathon and get over the finishing line). I had to overcome the sceptics.

'I have to tell you how great it was for me. I work at a laundry and there is a machine for repairs, and as I was losing weight my trousers kept getting bigger and bigger and the lady who ran the machine kept hacking away at them. My pockets, that had once been on the side of my pants ended up being my back pockets, side by side!! I have got rid of all my fat clothes, as I'll never, never go back to them again.

'The diet works, providing you have the determination to make it work for you. You've got to set your mind on it and change your life. Make a goal you are going to win.

'And when people tell you that you look marvellous and wonderful for the first time in years it becomes the motivation to keep you going. I know that I must be rigid – I can put on weight easily and I can't allow it to ever gain up on me again. If I want to keep the way I am now I must accept the fact I have a new life and must adopt new eating habits.

'I don't have to stay religiously sole source forever, but I do keep an eye on what is happening on the scales and if I start seeing an increase – I start that very day – to cut out a meal or two.

'At first, I used to do it week by week, but for me that was a mistake. I gained back a little weight. So now every morning I get on the scales and if I have gone up a bit that day I go straight on the diet sole source.

'While the people around me at home and at work have colds and flu' one after another, I have only had "half a cold" in over a year. I've had no time off from work for illness whatsoever and I guess I've become a bit boastful about it (sort of like a reformed smoker). I tell everyone they need to get their weight off and get fit and have better nutrition. I've become quite critical now that I realize what I used to feel like and look like. I want everyone to become more educated about it.

'Sure, I hear all the stories of "Oh, my whole family has always been overweight," or "I've got gland trouble," they just don't get my sympathy. All the story really is, is that they eat more than their body requires. I'm grateful for my new life! I'd be glad to tell everyone of my success!!'

CHAPTER SEVEN

THE CAMBRIDGE COUNSELLOR

The Inspiration

In the early spring of 1980, Clara McDermott was forty-eight years old, 5 ft 6 in. (167 cm) tall and weighed a hefty 196 lbs (14 st.; 89 kg). She was a 'professional' yo-yo dieter of some 20 years, with first-hand experience of every diet that came on the market. She would lose a little and gain it right back again.

Clara had a very successful wig and dress shop in Salt Lake City, Utah, but she had begun to hate herself and the way she looked. What most frightened her, though, was what was happening to her health. Working in the shop, climbing stairs, or just walking, began getting harder and harder and her blood pressure was dangerously high.

One day she noticed a headline in a weekly newspaper – 'The Incredible Diet'. She bought a copy, read about the research and the very low calories and felt she might finally have come across a diet that could work for her. She promptly sent off for a four-week supply.

In two months she had lost 56 lbs (25 kg) and her friends and customers became so excited at how wonderful and healthy she was looking that they began totally disrupting her work in the shop. They were always wanting to know how she lost so much weight and why after losing it she wasn't saggy and gaunt-looking. She finally began handing out mail-order forms for the Cambridge Diet, but then these people would telephone her and ask questions and for advice on how to use the product. They also couldn't wait to tell her of their own successful experiences.

In time, she could see that it would make better sense to buy the Cambridge Diet in large enough quantities to supply the demand, but she found she still spent all her time explaining and answering questions. Clara already had a business to run and the addition of what seemed to be the beginning of yet another business was quite disturbing, so she announced that if they wanted to purchase the product and talk about the diet they could come to the shop on Thursdays at 6.30 p.m.

Soon there wasn't a room at the shop big enough to hold them all. You see, when you are successful at losing weight you catch the attention of all those who know you, and they too want to go on the diet. As you can understand, they wanted direct contact with someone who could answer their questions.

In this area of the United States the art of counselling others on their social and moral problems was already well established by members of the Church of Jesus Christ of Latter-Day-Saints (Mormons) to which Clara belongs. The Mormons believe in a healthy life and abstain from alcohol, coffee, tea and tobacco for this reason. However, one of the problems in their society is obesity, which is inconsistent with their aims. Therefore, Clara supplied the method she already knew about – counselling her patrons who wanted to know more about the Cambridge Diet.

Because of the size of her operation, individual attention was impossible and she therefore held weekly sessions, called 'Cambridge Meetings', at which she and others who had lost a lot of weight gave their testimonies and thereby motivated others to start the diet and continue. Those who had equal success also became counsellors and some of them, besides attending weekly meetings, advised each other over the telephone, swapping stories, motivating and generally keeping in touch

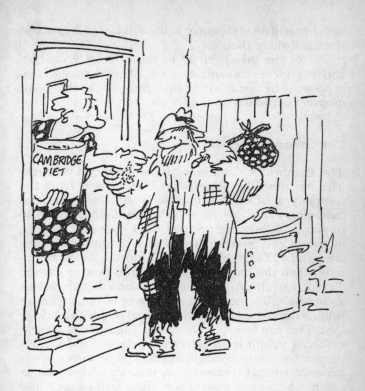

with others' progress.

It wasn't long before Clara was ordering close to $5,000 a week of Cambridge Diet and supplying nearly 800 people. Cambridge Plan International, who had their offices in Monterey, California, and at that time were still selling the diet by mail order, wondered how it was that one customer could be placing such large orders, and they contacted her. As a result of discussions with Clara and her husband Jim, the company originated the 'Founders' Circle' of 50 leaders in the spring of 1981 and thus began the counsellor system as it is today. Within six months, Clara and the counsellors with her had 50,000 people in the Salt Lake City area on the Cambridge Diet.

Out of the group of 50 in the original Founders' Circle grew an organization of 200,000 counsellors, supported by a staff of 1,000 employees at the head-quarters in Monterey, California.

The Counsellor System

The Cambridge Counsellor is an independent agent who has used the Cambridge Diet, buys it from the company at a basic wholesale price, and sells it to customers called 'patrons' for a profit. In addition to physically selling the product the Counsellor advises, motivates and generally liaises with patrons while they are using it. This is particularly important at the beginning when the patron is initiated into how to use the diet successfully. Anyone can purchase a diet product at a chemist's, but not many people read the literature fully or understand the full potential of the Cambridge Diet. This can be explained by the Counsellor.

Losing weight is an extremely personal and serious project for the overweight sufferer. The dieter needs personal contact, reassurance, praise and encourage-ment, compliments to raise their self-image, and constant motivation. The Counsellor is always available to listen and to provide an honest interest in the patron's progress. You can't buy personal contact off a chemist's shelf!

Self Example

Counsellors are those people who have successfully used the Cambridge Diet for weight loss or as a nutri-tional supplement. Because of their enthusiasm they want to share their success with others, and very quickly

82

they end up with a group of patrons to serve. Their only advertisement is themselves. Often their friends ask, 'How is it that you have lost so much weight?' and they reply, 'On this new diet.' 'What diet?' 'The Cambridge Diet.' 'What's that?' In no time at all the Counsellor has added a new patron to his or her list.

It is virtually impossible to sell the diet if you are overweight or at least have not lost a substantial amount of weight. To prove the diet works is the best advertisement there is, but of more importance is the effect on the Counsellors themselves. Many have lost weight on innumerable diets and regained it. A successful Cambridge business is the strongest inhibitor of weight regain that I know. The Counsellors have to prove to their patrons that in addition to rapid weight loss, it is possible to achieve the most elusive state of all, permanent weight maintenance.

The Cambridge Meeting

Encouraging people to start on the Cambridge Diet and to follow them up over several weeks is a time-consuming business. To use the time most efficiently and effectively the Counsellor organizes a weekly meeting, either at home or at a special meeting room in the vicinity. There, he or she can educate, instruct and demonstrate the virtues of the diet and answer any questions. A very important part of any meeting is to have patrons who have lost weight tell about their success. With such evidence before them it is rather rare for a potential patron to leave a Cambridge Meeting without purchasing at least one tin of the product.

Sponsoring

Counsellors are able to sponsor their own patrons to become Counsellors themselves, but before doing so, the Counsellor has to ensure that the patron has taken the product faithfully for a reasonable period of time, and that he or she is conversant with its proper use and seems competent enough to perform the duties of a Counsellor.

Within a few months a Counsellor may have quite a group of new Counsellors, of which he or she has become the originator or leader.

Group Leaders

When a total of 15 Counsellors has been established, the originator of the group can become a Group Leader, and then receives additional remuneration from the Company. In return it is the Counsellor's direct responsibility to look after and instruct all the other Counsellors. Also, these duties can be conveniently carried out at a Cambridge Meeting. The Group Leader will usually split the meeting into two parts. The first is for new patrons and the second is for the Counsellors he or she is supervising. To help in this task, the Group Leader organizes special seminars and workshops to keep all the Counsellors fully up to date with new products and the latest information on health education.

At seminars and conferences (which are organized by the company) the Group Leaders are fully educated in areas of nutrition and behaviour modification, support and motivation, how to deal with excessive weight loss and ways to work with health professionals. They are given an up-date on new products and future research. Tips on running a successful business are also provided. It is at these conferences that the company gives individual recognition to those Group Leaders who have excelled in sales, but most important, to those who have given their personal time and dedication to their patrons. The Group Leader then passes on the information to the Counsellors.

Safety

Many people do not read instructions or the small print on the side of packaging material well enough (if at all). A vital part of the Counsellor's job is to see that the patrons are fully conversant with safety regulations and aspects. These include the following points:

1 To advise the patron to see his or her doctor and discuss whether it is all right to start the diet. This is particularly important if a person is receiving medication or has a chronic medical condition.

2 To indicate that the Cambridge Diet can be used as a nutritional supplement, and that there are certain classes of individuals who should not use the diet as their sole source of nutrition. These are the very young, the elderly, pregnant and lactating women.

3 To advise that the diet should not be taken as a sole source of nutrition for more than four weeks at any one time unless under the constant care of a general practitioner.

4 To advise on minor side-effects.

5 To advise on how weight maintenance can be achieved using sound nutritional principles and help with ideas for recipes.

Health Education

Throughout the world, health authorities are concerned about the bad nutritional state of their populations. They know that coronary heart disease, high blood pressure, diabetes, cancer and many other diseases can be greatly reduced by an improvement in nutritional habits which I have discussed earlier, in Chapter 5. Governments often provide funds to educate the public through television and radio, and magazine and newspaper articles. As Chairman of the British Food Education Society I have a special interest in educating the public and in the past have written a number of leaflets and books and appeared on television programmes to this end. Despite heavy expenditure, the results have so far been disappointing. In Britain particularly, there has been little progress in changing the general public's eating habits compared with some other countries, such as Sweden, for example.

In general the Counsellors who sell the Cambridge Diet are people who believe in a good healthy life and they are encouraged not to be in the business just to sell the diet, but to educate people in better nutritional habits.

The Role of the Counsellor in Society

In practice the Counsellor system has proved very effective and offers society more than at first sight seems possible. There are innumerable facets to the contribution the Counsellor can make. Over the telephone he or she encourages the patrons in the same way that a sponsor in Alcoholics Anonymous or a Samaritan would. Many of the techniques used at the weekly meeting are similar to Weight Watchers or those of behavioural therapists.

Only those people who truly want to help and serve other people are successful at being Counsellors. You must care deeply about the welfare of those you are serving and make every effort to make them experience the benefits of good nutrition and successful weight loss – perhaps for the very first time in their lives.

CHAPTER EIGHT

THE PSYCHOLOGICAL APPROACH

Achieving success with the Cambridge Diet involves a great deal of psychology. The person who is trying to lose weight must appreciate that his or her psychological outlook on life will change. Counsellors, too, will be more successful if they have a basic knowledge of what psychological problems beset their patrons. The following pages give my views of how a good psychological approach to the use of the Cambridge Diet can help to produce a successful outcome for everyone.

Motivation

Success on the Cambridge Diet can be achieved only by a person who is well motivated. A typical example is the person who is impressed with a friend's new slim figure, and longs to copy his or her achievement. Persuaded to try the Diet, the new dieter finds the weight rolls off within a few days, and is so delighted that he or she perseveres.

On the other hand, there are many people who are not spontaneously motivated and are unwilling to start dieting. They are looking for an easy way of curing their problems and one which will make them lose weight. In their own opinion, they are the victims of being overweight and are not responsible for it. It is this type of person who gives all the excuses: 'I don't believe that the Cambridge Diet would work for me as I think that you must just eat sensibly', 'I'll try it as a supplement but I don't believe that 330 calories a day is enough', 'I can't go "Sole Source" for any more than one day, I have to have "Real Food".' This resistance can be countered if they can be persuaded to attend a Cambridge Meeting. They will then see that all their excuses are invalid.

Moderation

Another myth some people believe is that moderation works. The reason why they are usually overweight is because moderation *doesn't* work. If a piece of apple pie tastes wonderful, how many people can really leave it on a plate because there are too many calories in it, even though their conscience tells them that they are being excessive and immoderate and that the pie is fattening? Your experience tells you that it tastes good. And if you eat it all your hunger will disappear and you will feel full. If, on the other hand, you force yourself to stop eating because it contains too many calories, you will not feel satisfied. It is the old story, that whatever you are told you cannot have (even by your own mind) you still tend to want. People who fail on diets usually believe it is because they do not have enough willpower or are not counting their calories precisely enough, or are cheating. The idea that one can lose weight by just eating in moderation is false. For most people moderation is fine for maintaining their weight, and preventing it from going up, but not for losing it in the first place.

The great strength of the Cambridge Diet plan in losing weight is that the person does not have to make a choice in how much food to eat, it is already worked out for them – just three Cambridge meals a day. There are no further decisions to be made.

Behavioural Therapy

Extensive psychological research has shown that many overweight patients have a different eating style from people of normal weight or those who are thin. During a single meal overweight individuals may consume the same number of calories but they may eat them more quickly. The overweight take larger mouthfuls of food and chew their food less and drink far more with their meals. In general the obese person does not eat to satisfy hunger, but responds to food 'cues'. These 'cues' are anything around them which trigger off the desire to eat. For instance, what time of day it is, sitting and watching TV, the sight of food or even a food advert.

The psychology of fat people in relation to food appears to be quite different from that of people who are thin. Based on these observations, Dr Richard Stuart developed what he called 'Behavioural Therapy For Obesity'. It is based on training the overweight to resist food cues and to change their eating patterns. Those interested are recommended to read his book (see Bibliography).

A number of obesity experts have been interested in combining the Cambridge Diet with behavioural therapy. Obviously, it applies only at meal-times and when the Diet is being used as a nutritional supplement. During a period of sole source, food cues become less sharp and it is possible for a dieter to prepare food for other people and to resist the temptation to eat while doing so. If behavioural therapy is to be of any use at all it is during a weight maintenance programme.

The Cambridge Diet and Behaviour

In my experience I have found that taking the Cambridge Diet changes the dieter's whole mental attitude to food and eating. The person who has lost a lot of weight taking the Cambridge Diet as sole source tends only to eat when food is delicious and he or she is truly hungry. It is only natural that such people should take their time over what they are eating and concentrate on it and enjoy it. They remember what a struggle it was to lose all the weight and how they had to abandon ordinary food completely. It was tough! For this reason, people on the weight maintenance programme become very selective about what they eat and when they eat.

Although the advantages of behavioural therapy can be thoroughly recommended, for most people it will eventually be doing what comes naturally and reinforce what is in fact, common sense. The food cues, which triggered off their eating before they went on the diet, often disappear, because at long last they have much more control over themselves.

Personality Types

In my own contact with patients at the Obesity Clinic at Addenbrooke's Hospital, Cambridge, I find that there seem to be four main types of overweight people:

1 *The Junkaholics* – These people become overweight because of bad eating habits. They eat too much food of poor nutritional value, consisiting mainly of fat, sugar and alcohol. They are the 'Junk Food Addicts' who, besides eating at mealtimes, eat snacks continuously and become overweight purely because of force of habit or social reasons. Their main problem is lack of education about good nutrition.

2 *The Socializers* – These people become overweight because of professional or social reasons. They have to attend innumerable business lunches, dinners, cocktail parties and receptions. Their consumption of alcohol is often excessive and the good food

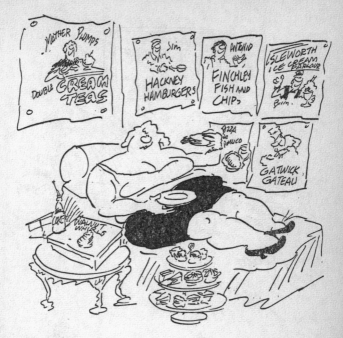

The Junkaholics

provided for them tempts them to eat more than they need. Many business executives, MPs, college professors and celebrities come into this category.

3   *The Metabolics* – These are people who need very little food because their metabolism is set very low and they need very little energy for normal daily life. Often such people require only 800 calories, or less, per day and if they take in more than this they gain weight. Usually, these people have been overweight since they were young and come from families in which the mother or father have also been overweight.

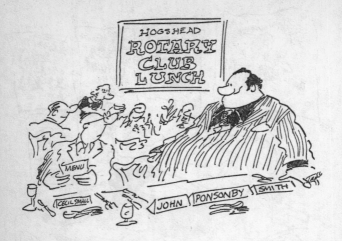

The Socializers

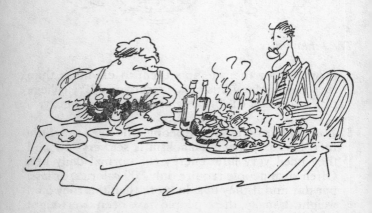

The Metabolics

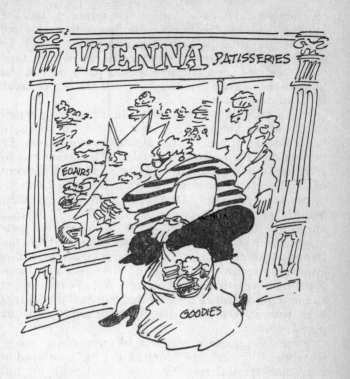

The Bingers

4 *The Bingers* – This group of people are overweight because they take refuge in eating to solve their social problems, and to soothe themselves from stress. They often go on eating 'binges'. These are the truly psychologically abnormal. In a way, they are addicted to food, especially carbohydrates, in the same way that an alcoholic is addicted to alcohol.

Within our population it is difficult to determine what are the proportions of the different types categorized above. Perhaps a clue can be given in that the greatest proportion of overweight people in our society is to be found in the lower socio-economic classes. In other words it is the poor who become overweight. One could perhaps speculate that they become overweight because they have less money to spend and buy cheaper foods of poor nutritional value.

In my early days of research, when I was concerned chiefly with trying to produce a model for coronary heart disease in rats, I coincidentally came across the perfect diet for making rats obese. The secret was to give them a normal diet to which was added 40 per cent of fat. This could be any type of fat, but in our experiments we used butter. After a few months the animals became enormously obese, so that it was virtually impossible for them to move off the bottom of their cages. About 60 per cent of their calories came from fat. In our population the average is about 40 per cent. The interesting feature of the diet of these rats was that it contained everything they needed, but in order to get all the required nutrients they had to eat all the fat that went with it. I suspect that it is the same with our population.

Some fat people are rather like my obese rats — searching for nutrients! Much of the foods offered in supermarkets and restaurants is loaded with fat and refined sugar. In order to get all the nutrients needed, vast quantities of calories have to be consumed.

Of course the psychologist might argue that obese people are so stressed and unhappy that they would naturally seek solace in eating, and that this is why they become fat. Overweight in my rats was not caused by stress. Animals of a similar age, but fed on a normal non-fatty rat cake, were all very lean and healthy. If the stress of living in a cage had been the reason for their being overweight, all the rats would have been fat.

I am convinced that most of the obesity in Western-style countries is caused by faulty nutrition and that the majority of people come into Class 1 – my 'Junkaholic' category. The other three categories occur less frequently in the general population, but do accumulate in the obesity clinics of university hospitals because they are the most difficult cases for ordinary doctors to treat.

Success Ratings

Not one can fail to lose weight if the Cambridge Diet is used *as directed*, and this applies to all classes of over-weight person, whichever psychological category is relevant. However, the ease with which an individual of each psychological type can be encouraged to lose weight varies tremendously.

The greatest success can be achieved among the 'Junkaholics'. For them it is purely a process of education. They will lose weight very quickly and reach their ideal weight within a few months, because in general they are only about 30-40 lbs (13-18 kg) overweight. Their main problem is weight maintenance. Unless a change of eating habits can be established they will rapidly regain their weight to what it was before dieting began. One way this can be prevented is by their using the Cambridge Diet three times daily as a nutritional supplement and combining it with supplementary food of modest calorie content, based on sound nutritional principles.

The 'Socializers' are more difficult to help because they are usually unable to find a period long enough to undergo sole source dieting. It is socially unacceptable at present to attend a public dinner and present your glass of Cambridge as a substitute. During the course of a year, however, there may be a lull in social activities and many 'Socializers' attempt sole source nutrition during their holidays. Weight maintenance is relatively easy. It means using the social events as the main food supply. During the rest of the time ordinary meals are replaced by the Cambridge Diet. It is also helpful for them to reduce their alcohol consumption and drink mineral water instead. Success is variable but many 'Socializers' are intelligent people and can work out a permanent solution for themselves.

The people I call 'Metabolics' have a real problem. Throughout their lives they have a continual struggle to keep their weight down and more often than not, they are massively obese despite a low calorie intake. Weight loss for them, even on the Cambridge Diet is painstakingly slow, with innumerable plateaus. Usually they are well motivated dieters, and it is clearly a question of perseverance, so that they can eventually reach their ideal weight. Once there, they are condemned for life to about 800 to 1,000 calories per day – or even less. However, with the Cambridge Diet providing 330 calories they can easily survive on one 'reasonable' meal per day of 400 to 500 calories. It takes considerable willpower for these people, but their zeal and determination usually wins, and they become proud of their good looks and better health.

The 'Bingers' present a very difficult problem indeed. First of all it is difficult to motivate them to start dieting. Having done so they usually fall by the wayside, because their problem is not just bad eating habits or being overweight by misfortune. Other psychological factors are involved. Unless they can get to grips with their problems, identify the reasons for their addiction to food, and overcome them, then there is litle long-term hope. Such people present a real challenge to the doctor or Counsellor.

The approach to the 'Binger' is much the same as to anyone addicted to alcohol or any other drug. The individual has to admit the addiction and 'kick' the habit. Unfortunately, complete abstinence is impossible! Food is vital to our survival and if we don't have food we die. This, however, is where the Cambridge Diet can make a difference. To the 'Binger', the

Cambridge Diet is not 'real' food, it is food replacement. Using it, he can 'kick' the habit and get over the withdrawal symptoms without being ill.

A number of 'Bingers' have lost a great deal of weight on the diet, but the long-term outlook is poor.

Sexual Relationships and Weight Loss

In our society, erroneously or not, everyone believes that being slim is more attractive than being fat. This can be the source of some psychological problems which have come to light with extensive use of the Cambridge Diet. When the overweight person diets successfully, a new body image is imposed on him or her. More often than not that person suddenly becomes sexually attractive. Perhaps for the first time in her life, a rather plain, fat girl has become so attractive that the opposite sex begins to pay attention to her. If she is not accustomed to this type of sexual 'head turning', it can be extremely upsetting, especially to someone who has lived a very sheltered life. Her parents may have taught her to avoid being 'too attractive' to the opposite sex since it could be 'dangerous'. It may be too difficult for her to cope with the new situation and she may be so worried by it that she will intentionally regain her earlier weight.

Needless to say, this is an unusual situation but one that happens. It requires careful counselling to enable her to come to terms with herself. Success can only be achieved by convincing her that there is nothing to be ashamed of in possessing this lovely new body and eventually to enjoy the excitement of her new sexual attractiveness.

Difficult situations do not just apply to females. One of our patients reported that his wife actually told him that he looked haggard and old. This was completely false as his appearance had tremendously improved and he had already reported that the girls at the office had begun taking an interest in him. But his wife was worried that she might lose him and tried everything she could to spoil his new self-confidence. Fortunately, he was able to recognize the problem and reassure his wife of his love and fidelity, so that she eventually accepted the situation.

An enormous physical change in one partner can create havoc in a 'reasonably' happy marriage in a different way. Many women and men who are overweight find it difficult to attract a partner and sometimes settle for 'second best'. Perhaps they have little in common, but will marry anyway. On losing weight and becoming more physically attractive, the man or woman begins to feel cheated by life and loses interest in their partner and subsequently the marriage. The partner then feels threatened and encourages the newly slim partner to regain the weight so that the feeling of safety will return. Instead of feeling enormously proud of the successful partner, jealousy and insecurity prevail. This can eventually lead to the break-up of the marriage unless the pair find a way of reassuring each other of their love for each other.

One of our patients lost about 100 lbs (45 kg) and had become quite a beautiful woman. In the end neither she nor her husband were able to handle the change in her appearance and both ended up having extra-marital affairs. They were trying to sort out the insecurities that this change had brought into their lives. Eventually she regained about 40 pounds and unfortunately, although they remain married to one another, their lives are now overshadowed with insecurity and distrust. It's sad that this does happen, but possibly the situation could be avoided by counselling husbands and wives on the possible psychological repercussions of weight loss.

Similar situations have been reported by Alcoholics Anonymous with regard to alcoholism. It sometimes happens that when an alcoholic stops drinking the family is unable to accept the 'new' person because they felt a kind of security in being 'superior'.

Fortunately, weight loss most often leads to very happy endings! The following story is more typical. One of our very successful patients was enormously obese, weighing 21 stone (294 lbs; 133 kg). She and her husband had married while she was fat. After 11 months she had successfully shed 11 stone (154 lbs; 70 kg). You don't have to ask her husband if he is proud of her. All you have to do is to see his face when they are together! He literally beams at the sight of his slim, beautiful 'new' wife. He enjoys her success and likes to tell everybody how much money it has cost him just to outfit her with a new wardrobe, and then with a twinkle in his eye he confides what fun it has been and how his biggest thrill was getting her into a slinky bikini!!

The Last Few Pounds/Kilos

It is a common experience for some people to plateau just short of their target weight. Many of them start off following the Cambridge Diet correctly and quickly experience dramatic results. They begin to look and feel better and are proud of their progress. Their friends notice how slim they are looking and ask what was the reason for their success. Then something very curious happens. Just when they are about to get down to their ideal weight, they either plateau or put weight on, which means that they are not following the diet as they should. Often they make excuses, claiming to be a victim of a bad cold or of being depressed. One psychologist suggests that the reason is that some people are fearful of achieving their goal – ideal weight loss. If they were to achieve it there would be no further challenges for them.

On the other hand, it could be explained by a loss of motivation. One lady, who had been severely overweight and successfully shed much of the excess, became rather 'big headed' by all the fuss made over her. Whenever she looked at her 'before' photographs she could see what tremendous progress she had made. Then, someone she hadn't seen for a long time came along and went into raptures about how much she had changed and how wonderful she looked. As a result, a sense of self-satisfaction settled in and that was the end of her desire and motivation to continue to lose weight.

Whatever the explanation, everyone is unanimous that the last few pounds/kilos are certainly the hardest!

CHAPTER NINE

IS IT WORTHWHILE?

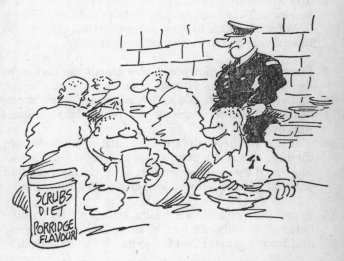

SCRUBS DIET PORRIDGE FLAVOUR

If you are severely overweight and have lost pounds
and pounds to achieve your ideal weight, you will have
found the going tough. While the Cambridge Diet is
easy to use and a sure way of achieving success, it needs
high motivation and a lot of grit and determination to
continue month after month. For those who were
moderately overweight or had just a small amount to
lose it was easier, but still required a high degree of
motivation. Is all the trouble worth it? And will the

long-term benefits be easily apparent? Let's look at some of the positive benefits you will achieve:

1 There is a feeling of great achievement to have solved finally what for many years has been an extremely difficult problem – the loss of that unwanted weight. All the emotional and physical problems caused by that undesired fat will have disappeared, one hopes, for ever.

2 You will be astonished at how youthful and attractive you look. Your friends and relatives will comment on it. You will be able to dress in more stylish clothes and have a very much improved body image.

3 From a medical viewpoint, you are almost certain to live longer. Your risk of coronary heart disease, diabetes, or high blood pressure are very much reduced because you have reached a normal, ideal weight.
   If any of these diseases have afflicted you before dieting, the symptoms may have been very much improved by your weight loss. The chances are that you will be able to live a longer and healthier life.

4 From the physical viewpoint, you will feel much better. You will sleep less, be more active and athletic and have a greater zest for living life to its fullest.

5 Your social life will be improved. No longer will it be embarrassing for you to appear in public as perhaps it was in the past. Instead of avoiding people you will make an increasing circle of new friends and acquaintances, purely because you are not hiding yourself away from life and public gaze.

6 You will be much better off financially, too. Fewer days off work because of illness, the continual taking

of the Cambridge Diet as a nutritional supplement will ensure that you feel well, are able to work harder and thus have better prospects of earning more.

From every point of view it is well worth it!!

The following story is a good illustration of one young lady who discovered exactly what these benefits meant to her.

Personal Story of Christine Baynham, Greenford, Middlesex

'When I married in 1980 I got my weight down to 9½ stone (133 lbs; 60 kg) for the wedding. Soon after we were married I was cooking a great deal and I began to put on weight. When I became pregnant in 1982 my weight shot up to 15 stone (210 lbs; 95 kg) during the pregnancy. After I had my baby I was 13 st. 2(184 lbs; 83.5 kg). I tried dieting myself by eating sensibly, but I probably got too many calories for my metabolic rate. It took 18 months to lose 13 lbs (6 kg). I finally got down to 12 st. 3 (171 lbs; 77.5 kg). I didn't feel at all well and had no energy at all. I found I just wasn't coping with a small baby and my housework, ironing, etc. It was such a great effort! I was suffering migraines and my skin was terrible.

'About this time I began to have a lot of depression. I wouldn't even go out of the house because I thought people were looking at me. Life became terrible for my little girl because she wasn't getting any fresh air at all.

'My mother began to feel I was "going a little bit funny". If someone came to the door I wouldn't let them in. I continually felt that people were staring at me and putting me down. She was wondering if it really was just because I was overweight or if I was truly "going odd". Well it was my weight! I was walking around in my maternity clothes and I was ashamed.

103

Neighbours and friends would ask if I was pregnant again – of course I wasn't! Here I was, looking like I was expecting another one there and then.

'This really affected our social life. I wouldn't go to any parties or if we would get invitations at Christmas or New Year, I'd make excuses not to go. I'd say the baby couldn't be left with grandparents or a child minder. I also felt embarrassed about my clothes. Everybody else was in nice party clothes or tight leather trousers and I had no interest in the clothes I could get into. They were old fashioned. Here I was, a young person, in dresses for a lady about forty.

'My husband wasn't a whole lot of help because he said he loved me any way I was. He said it was my personality that was important. Heavy or thin, it didn't make any difference to him. But it made a difference to me! I felt I wasn't good enough for him. I was ashamed when he would introduce me to his friends and I would hang back so he wouldn't have to say I was his wife.

'During this time my mum went on the Cambridge Diet and lost about 50 lbs (22 kg). She then introduced me to her Cambridge Counsellor. I started the Cambridge Diet on 23 April, 1984 weighing 12 st. 3 (171 lbs; 77.5 kg). I was preparing meals for my husband and little girl and I found I had to drink my Cambridge Diet while I was cooking their meals and when they ate I would go upstairs and have a bath or read a book. I needed to get out of the room. This lasted for just a little while, but when I saw I had lost a stone (6 kg) in two weeks I knew it was going to work for me. From then on I could fix potatoes or any kind of food and it didn't bother me at all.

'Then I began to notice I had a lot more energy! I was pushing the baby in her pram or push chair (something I had hardly ever done before; everything was done in the car).

'By my fifth week I started to attend a keep-fit class for mothers and daughters. This was run by my health visitor and she was so surprised to see me out of the house and being active. Then I started swimming and jogging. People began to say my skin looked so much better and wasn't I losing weight or something. I also began to notice that I no longer had headaches any more.

'I continued to lose about 16 lbs (7 kg) a month. By 10 August 1984 I weighed 8 st. 10 (122 lbs; 55 kg). A loss of 50 lbs (22 kg) in 3½ months! I had been wearing a size 20 dress and mac and could finally get into a size 10. I am taking the diet three meals a day now and adding one light meal of other foods to maintain my weight.

'My husband and I ran into a bit of a problem at first. He went through a "jealousy stage". If I spoke with the butcher he wanted to know what was funny and what we were talking about (how to cook the cut of meat, of course!) When the phone rang he would hang around the phone and ask, "Who was that"? "What did they want"? It has now worn off a bit. I guess he's seen that I'm not going to run off with anyone and that I still love him.

'My personality has really changed completely. I actually went and applied for a job at British Airways for a part-time Ground Hostess. When I got there I found 80 other girls also applying. They were all so glamorous, well dressed with lovely make-up. After reading the application form I could see that I couldn't afford to take the job as the salary was too low, but it made me feel so good to know I would even go out and apply for a job along with girls who looked as they did. Anyway, I went ahead and stayed for the interview. I kept thinking, "I'm just as good as they are"! Before, I wouldn't have even considered going for such a job.

'Since then I have been reinstated as a Clerical Officer, part-time, until my daughter goes to school and then I will go full-time. This is quite a change from the girl who was hiding at home, refusing to see people, who wouldn't go on holiday. (Oh, by the way, we have

105

just booked a holiday and I know I can wear a bikini on the beach without any embarrassment now.)

'I have a lot of ambitions now. My husband says he can't keep up with me and with what I am doing, but he says he is very pleased. I guess he just doesn't know what to expect of me any more with my new energy and improved self-image.

'Thanks to the Cambridge Diet I now have everything going for me and I know I can keep the weight off and stay this way!'

Christine has now herself become a Cambridge Counsellor.

PART II
The Cambridge Discovery

CHAPTER TEN

THE PERFECT FOOD

In the United States and the United Kingdom tens of thousands now take their 'Cambridge' every day, either for weight maintenance or just as a delicious, healthy, nutritional supplement. It has become an acceptable food like Cornflakes or Mars bars.

For those who are overweight, complete nutrition is obtainable in only 330 calories. All the major ingredients are natural and the Diet consists of common foodstuffs, fortified with synethetic vitamins, minerals and trace elements. I consider that the Cambridge Diet is the perfect food for many of us, from a nutritional point of view. There is no food naturally obtainable that contains all known nutrients in so few calories.

Much of our knowledge about the importance of many nutrients in our diet arises from agricultural research. A great deal more money has been spent on the nutrition of farm animals than on that of human beings. For many years, animal feeds have been supplemented and fortified with additional vitamins and minerals. As a result, the animals are fitter and healthier, milk yields are larger and the carcases contain more protein.

My first job as a young scientist at the Dunn Nutrition Laboratory, Cambridge, was to prepare a nutritionally complete diet for guinea pigs. The diet, in fact, consisted of a mixture of clearly defined foodstuffs, such as milk protein, starch and oil, fortified with all the known vitamins and minerals. The guinea pigs thrived on it, and their growth rate was very much better than on their 'natural' diet of oats and bran. During my stay at this laboratory, tons of the new diet were used in our experiments. One day I remarked to one of my assistants, 'I wonder if we as human beings will ever eat such a terrible concoction?' He laughed and said, 'I hope not!'

My nutritional training in those early days was of enormous benefit later on, in formulating the Cambridge Diet. The guinea pig diet was always in the back of my mind. Maybe it wasn't such a terrible concoction as we thought. The guinea pigs certainly liked it. Flavoured with vanilla, strawberry or chocolate, it is possible that many people would have found it acceptable and enjoyable. Indeed it is very curious that the perfect foodstuff has never been developed before – just for nutrition. There are a few foods on the market enriched with vitamins and minerals, but most of these have a number of defects. Usually, they do not contain *everything* necessary, and their calorie content is too high. Quite often they are meant only for sick people, and their palatability leaves much to be desired. What has happened by chance is that, though originally intended for slimming, the Cambridge Diet has become accepted by many people as a staple food in its own right. By taking the Cambridge Diet, we can receive all the benefits of complete nutrition in a very palatable form, just as farm animals have been doing for years.

Many varieties of the Cambridge Diet, available as soups and milk shakes, are made by fortifying milk and soya products. However, there is no reason why any mixture of foods could not be similarly fortified. In present day society, many people consume what nutritionists term 'junk food', particularly snack foods and confectionery. There is no reason why junk food should not be fortified to make it nutritious too. In fact this has been done now, for Cambridge chocolate bars already exist. In my opinion it is much better to feed people what they like to eat, rather than to persuade them to eat other kinds of nutritious food which they don't particularly care for. I can see nothing wrong with a nutritious chocolate bar, as nutritious 'junk food' is certainly better than poor nutrition.

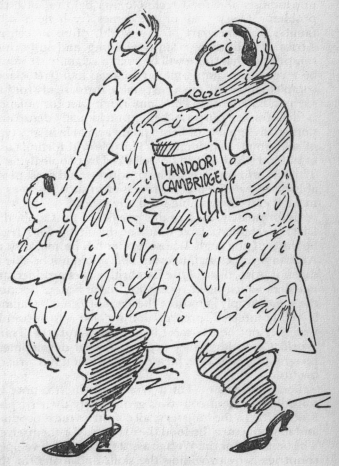

The Third World

While the chief concern of industrialized nations is to avoid over-consumption of food, much of the Third World is undernourished and starving. How can we as nutritionists and food technologists help to solve the problem? Every year or so, comes fresh news of a famine in some part of the world, often in central Africa. Usually there is ample warning, and authorities can predict that there will be such a calamity. It would be a relatively simple matter to keep handy stocks of complete foodstuffs in a very stable form, ready for just such an emergency. The Cambridge Diet formulation is ideal for the purpose, being nutritionally dense and potentially capable of being made available in any type of solid food. I envisage the Third World formula as a solid food which would be well liked by people living in Third World countries. The product would most probably be cereal-based and processed in such a way as to make it extremely stable for many years.

Unfortunately, most of the varieties of the Cambridge Diet at present available would be unsuitable for Africa, because of the high lactose content. The majority of Africans are lactose intolerant and would not be able to digest it. Also, most of the Cambridge Diet products are powders which need reconstituting in water. Because the water supply in most of the areas affected by famine is highly infected, presentation in such a form would probably not be the most beneficial. Thus, the Third World Cambridge Diet needs a special development programme, and I am pleased to say that it has already begun.

The problems of Third World nutrition cannot be solved by affluent countries giving away their surplus foodstuffs. In the long term all countries must produce and manufacture the food they require for themselves. The best way for the West to assist the under-developed countries is by providing the skills and loans for the

Buy two weeks' supply and get £2 off.

To take advantage of this great money-saving offer, simply complete, tear out and post this card off to us today - no stamp needed.

We will then send you, by return, a voucher entitling you to a £2 discount on the cost of two weeks' supply of the unique Cambridge Diet, together with full details on how to contact your local Cambridge Counsellor for both advice and supplies of the diet.

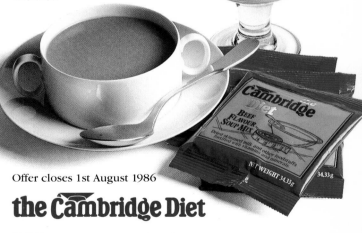

Offer closes 1st August 1986

the Cambridge Diet

NAME

ADDRESS

POSTCODE   TELEPHONE

I.D. No

Business reply service
Licence No. NC 698

Cambridge Nutrition Ltd.,
69-75 Thorpe Road,
Norwich,
Norfolk,
NR1 1BR.

manufacture of nutritional supplements, and
with local experts about which type of crops w
most suitable. The new staple food should be proce
from locally-grown cereals and protein, fortified
make a partial, or even a complete, life supporting diet
in famine-stricken areas. The necessary large stocks
could be stored in a manner similar to what is done in
Mormon storehouses.

For religious reasons, Mormons are taught to keep a
year or two of food in storage, to be used during time of
sudden calamity or disaster. They are taught this principle in order to provide for themselves and not to
become dependent on others. Many of these people
choose the Cambridge Diet because of its stability and
nutritional content. The church also maintains large
storehouses, where its needy members may obtain
supplies during a crisis. They are then obliged to
donate their time at these storehouses as a form of
repayment.

Third World nutrition comes high on the list of
priorities of the British charity I have set up, called the
Howard Foundation, which receives a major part of the
royalties from sales of the Cambridge Diet. It is an
enormous problem which no single organization will
ever be able to solve on its own. However, I believe that
the research which has gone into developing the
Cambridge Diet has a major contribution to make in
meeting the world's most important and urgent nutritional challenge. How those ten years of research were
started, with the aim of alleviating the misery and
disease endured by many fat people in the rich, over-
fed nations of the world, is a story which has its roots in
my own personal experience.

CHAPTER ELEVEN

THE RESEARCH

My interest in obesity began, as it has done for many others, from a personal need to lose weight. At the age of thirty I found myself fat and unhealthy. I had read books on diets and became an 'expert' on ways to lose weight. Nothing seemed to work for me. I did find it very easy to lose about 5-10 lbs (2-4 kg) and then the 'yo-yo' syndrome began making me fatter and fatter. So I decided to accept the challenge of creating a better treatment for the overweight, using myself as a guinea pig.

My first attempt was the commercial introduction – with a local milling company – of a very high protein slimming loaf, which was made from vegetables but had the same protein content as steak – at half the price! The idea was that people could eat as much of this loaf as they liked, and eventually, because it would stem their appetite, they would eat less. Altogether, with additional food, I was eating about 1,000 calories per day. In the short term it worked quite well for me and quite a few others. In a group of patients supervised by local general practitioners, patients lost about 10-15 lbs (4-6 kg), although it took several months to achieve it.

Through the press publicity about this loaf, I achieved a certain notoriety and was often asked to speak at public and scientific meetings. While I was not exactly thrilled by the results, at least this early work was sufficient to stimulate me to further and better research.

At this time, in the early 1960s, there were very few

scientists working on problems of the overweight and there was no scientific society where people interested in research could meet and discuss their results. With a group of friends, a steering committee was formed which eventually established the Association for the Study of Obesity. This still meets several times a year at the Royal Society of Medicine in London.

As a first step to getting the new association off the ground, I accepted the responsibility of organizing a conference on obesity in London in 1968 and delegated myself to summarize and review the latest treatments of obesity by means of diet. This involved a great deal of reading. To my amazement I found that in the past ten years many physicians had given up using food diets and had resorted to complete starvation – the Zero Calorie Diet – as the most effective way of producing weight loss. I was not very happy with what I read. The diet could only be used by patients in hospital and then it had one very major side effect, a very serious one – DEATH! There were at least five publications recording death in a number of patients treated by complete starvation. Mostly they were from cardiac problems, including severe degeneration of the heart muscle. It was quite clear that starvation really could not be used because of the high risk. Nevertheless, I was very impressed with the magnificent weight losses achieved. For instance, in one large trial men lost 35 lbs (16 kg) and women lost 26 lbs (11 kg). Other studies showed that people could lose as much as 70 lbs (31.75 kg) in 3½ months.

The decision to Collaborate

One of my colleagues on the Management Committee of the Association for the Study of Obesity was Dr Ian McLean Baird, of the West Middlesex Hospital, London. He acted as Chairman. He was one of the most influen-

115

tial and best respected physicians in the field, having already published a great deal on the health risk of obesity and on its high incidence in the British population. Being a London physician he also had access to hospital beds for research. He indicated that should I ever come up with a good idea he would be glad to collaborate. Like me, he saw that the combination of a nutritionist with experience in obesity research and a good all-round physician would make a strong team.

A year or so after the symposium, when we were dealing with the proceedings of the First National Meeting on Obesity, I discussed with Dr McLean Baird the subject of the Zero Calorie Diet. I had been impressed with the weight losses and the ability of the patients to stick to what must have been a ghastly regime — water and vitamin tablets. Surely, I speculated, there must be some nutritional formulation that could be devised with fewer calories than conventional diets (which at that time were about 800 calories) and yet provide sufficient nutrients to be safe. He agreed.

And so, in 1970, Dr McLean Baird and I decided to collaborate on developing the perfect diet which we hoped would have all the properties of a complete starvation regime, in that it would produce excellent weight loss, but would also be free from side effects, and certainly would *not* result in the death of the patient.

The Key to the Problem

The literature on the subject at that time was very sparse. Some work had been done in the 1930s on food diets of about 400 to 500 calories, but they had been virtually forgotten. No one knew if they were safe for the very long periods needed to treat severely obese patients. The key to the problem was to find out why death had occurred in patients using the complete starvation diet and then to come up with ways of preventing it. One young girl, who had been on a Zero Calorie Diet for over six months, died with damage to her heart muscle. Autopsy revealed her heart to be very thin and severely damaged, due, it was thought, to the absence of protein in the diet, so that her tissues had wasted during the course of the treatment. Thus, it was clear that the safe diet had to ensure that protein losses from the body were very small, otherwise damage could be done to the vital organs, such as heart, liver and lungs.

Protein losses can be determined by measuring nitrogen excretion in the urine and stools. If the amount of nitrogen excreted is greater than the intake, there is a 'negative nitrogen balance'. Our aim was to achieve, if possible, nitrogen equilibrium – that is, when the amount of nitrogen excreted is equal to that taken in. However, as we were to discover later, this is a theory which cannot be put into practice. When a person becomes overweight, about 9 per cent of the increase in body weight is due to protein, which of course has to be lost on weight reduction. Fortunately, in recent years, the amount of this additional protein has been accurately determined, and it is possible to allow for its contribution in the calculations.

The other danger in complete starvation is the excessive loss of electrolytes – such as sodium and potassium. Without sufficient potassium, the heart develops abnormal rhythms and can 'fibrillate', which means that the heart beats so fast that eventually the person dies of a heart attack. Although most physicians using the Zero Calorie Diet added electrolytes and vitamins, this was not always done, and it was quite clear that in some cases the patient had suffered from deficiency of essential items. Any diet, to be safe, has to contain all the vitamins, minerals and trace elements.

People in conditions of complete starvation within a few days develop 'ketosis'. This is due to the incomplete combustion of fat in which certain chemicals, called ketones, accumulate in the blood and eventually spill over into the urine. In a normal diet, the presence of carbohydrate enables the fat to be broken down completely, leaving no detectable ketones in the blood and urine. Ketones have a very similar effect on the brain to alcohol. In small doses they make people feel good, happy and euphoric. In large doses, however, they can, like alcohol, have severe disadvantages, making the person feel aggressive, out of sorts and unwell. It was obvious that we had to find the critical amount of carbohydrate necessary to give a *small* level of ketones, which would be beneficial to the patient and produce a feeling of well being. Before we started, this quantity was unknown. Carbohydrate is also important as a medium for retaining sodium and potassium in the body. Thus, inclusion of carbohydrates in the diet also stems the loss of these important electrolytes.

To summarize, we had to find the correct quantity of protein to be included in the diet, so that nitrogen losses would be as small as possible and carbohydrate had to be included to prevent excessive ketosis and to retain electrolytes.

The Initial Plan

At first we decided to carry out some studies on patients at the West Middlesex Hospital using formula diets which would include all the known nutrients, vitamins, minerals, trace elements and essential fatty acids. We felt it was very important that the patients should be carefully monitored using a battery of clinical and laboratory examinations so as to establish if the formulas were safe or not.

Experimental trials started in June 1970. The first patients were chosen from a long waiting list. They were four women and one man, all severely overweight and all had tried relentlessly to lose weight on other diet plans but had failed to do so. Their weights ranged from 220-350 lbs (15st. 7; 100 kg – 25 st.; 159 kg), and they were in hospital from 21 weeks up to one year.

In order to determine the smallest amount of protein and carbohydrate consistent with safety, the patients were given a variety of different formulas, starting each new one every few weeks. In addition to vitamins, minerals, trace elements and essential fatty acids a mixture of amino acids were given instead of protein. This was originally formulated for use by astronauts, and was considered to be nutritionally equivalent to a perfect protein. At first, carbohydrate was omitted and only protein given in gradually increasing quantities. Later on, small quantities of carbohydrate were added in the form of maltodextrins, a breakdown product of starch. The results were quite astonishing. Very small amounts of carbohydrate were found to have a dramatic effect on how much protein the body needed. Only about 30 grams (one ounce) of carbohydrate was enough to cut the requirement of protein by half. It was immediately apparent that the perfect diet required a finely tuned balance of carbohydrate and protein and that the total number of calories needed was smaller than ever expected – a mere 200 to 300 calories per day.

After much juggling with different formulas, we found that the minimum amounts needed were: protein 15 grams per day and carbohydrate 30 to 45 grams per day. There were strong grounds for believing that diets containing such small quantities of nutrients were safe. Nitrogen losses were extremely small, as were also losses of very important minerals, such as sodium and potassium.

Our first five patients were delighted with their excellent weight losses which averaged more than 4 lbs (1.8 kg) a week throughout the whole study. At the end of the experiment they were in better health than when they started.

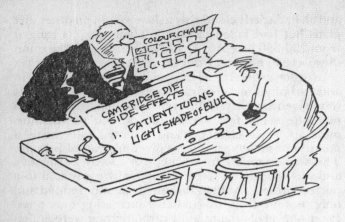

During the course of the trial we made some interesting conclusions, comparing the different dietary regimes. When receiving no calories at all, most of the patients felt very unwell, and spent most of their time in bed with headaches and muscle cramps. When they started getting a few calories they felt so much better that we could not keep them in their rooms. They became very active and spent a lot of time visiting and chatting to other patients at the hospital. So happy were they that special tasks around the hospital had to be found to keep their minds occupied.

The Second Trial

At this stage (in the summer of 1973) everything looked extremely promising, but to ensure that the diet was safe we had to experiment on a much larger group of patients. In the next trial we had as many as fifty patients. Our chief problem was the limited availability of hospital beds. To solve this problem patients were taken into hospital for only the first three weeks and were then seen as out-patients thereafter. While in hospital they got over their initial hunger pangs and became motivated to continue as out-patients. The safety of the diet was investigated throughout using a large number of laboratory tests, usually carried out at weekly intervals.

At this point, the diet was radically changed in protein content because the amino acid mixture proved much too expensive for use on a large scale. The new protein source chosen was an egg albumin. Many experts consider this to be the 'perfect protein', since it contains a balanced spectrum of amino-acids. In addition, the vitamins and minerals were included in the powder rather than giving them separately as a supplement.

Over the six month period, the average weight loss was 2½ lbs (1.1 kg) a week. At 18 weeks the average weight loss was 45 lbs (20 kg) – not bad, considering we were dealing with out-patients. The weight loss was, of course, not as great as we had seen in hospitalized patients. Quite a few of the out-patients completely dropped out and others obviously had found it very difficult to remain faithful to the programme. This was entirely understandable. The patients cheated because the mixture had a very unpleasant taste and it was more like taking a dose of medicine than food. There was no doubt in my mind that this concoction was much too unpalatable to present to the general public. People might try it for a short time but eventually they would give up. Nevertheless, these second trials (which lasted three years) were a huge success. None of the patients developed any significant abnormality while on the diet. They felt and looked well. We were convinced that we were on the right track.

A Question of Hunger

The major question was whether overweight people would ever be able to follow the course as out-patients without the initial hospitalization. We knew that it took a few days to get over the early hunger pangs and this might be too much for most people to tolerate. They would eventually cheat and not stick to the diet.

At this time (early 1975) a new appetite suppressant drug, Mazindol, had been released on to the market. It was claimed to be the most highly effective drug of its kind ever developed, without any side effects. The combination of this drug and our diet seemed ideal. We designed a study in which twenty patients took the new appetite suppressant while twenty others were given dummy tablets. Each group took its tablets for four weeks and then they changed over and took the other one instead. Quite early on in the trial it became clear which patients were taking the drug, because of the side-effects many of them suffered, such as nausea, sleep loss, palpitations and high euphoria. In some cases we had to stop the tablets altogether since the drug was so badly tolerated. It began to look as though the experiment would turn out to be a complete disaster. On analysing the results, however, we were quite amazed.

Those taking the appetite suppressant received no special benefits, and virtually everybody who consumed the diet, whatever the tablet they were given, lost weight. This was good news, as it showed that people could get over the initial feeling of hunger without the additional need of an appetite suppressant, with all the nasty side-effects. We found we could allow our patients to use the diet at home on an out-patient basis, rather than their being admitted to hospital.

Although we knew that in hospital the patients were not hungry when consuming the diet, it seemed incredible that the same could happen to out-patients. We had created the same lack of hunger (the medical term is 'anorexia') which occurs in complete starvation, yet the patients were able to live normal lives without the constraints of hospital. Our eight week study showed again that the regime was perfectly safe from the clinical viewpoint.

This breakthrough was what we had been looking for and provided the opportunity to carry out large numbers of studies on very many patients, not only in London but in Cambridge and elsewhere. Shortly afterwards, Professor Ivor Mills, Head of the Department of Medicine in Cambridge, agreed to set up the obesity clinic at Addenbrooke's Hospital at which I and one of his senior registrars saw thirty patients each week. This speeded up the development of the diet enormously.

The Cambridge Diet Appears

Before we started the next study we considered the protein source. We had found that there were several disadvantages in using egg albumin, even though it had high nutritional value. It was poor in taste and it would coagulate in hot drinks. It also proved to be expensive. In the spring of 1976 we turned instead to skimmed milk, which is an excellent source of casein and other milk proteins, and consulted with food technologists to work on the flavourings. Eventually, after a great deal of work, a 'not too unpalatable' complete diet was achieved. It contained 330 calories comprising 33 grams of protein, 44 grams of carbohydrate and 3 grams of fat. The flavours were chicken and asparagus soups and banana, peach, raspberry and strawberry drinks. This was to become the basis of the Cambridge Diet, which we hoped would be available eventually to millions of people.

It was important to examine the results of the next experiment carefully. We needed to check that the new formulation was safe, and this could only be done at the Metabolic Ward at the West Middlesex Hospital. Yet the ultimate use of the formulation was to be by outpatients. The obvious answer was a study in which we compared out-patients and in-patients. Altogether, a total of fifty obese patients were given the new flavoured formulation for from four to twelve weeks. After four weeks the mean weight loss was 20 lbs (9 kg) in hospitalized patients and 16 lbs (7.25 kg) in out-patients. After eight weeks both groups had lost a mean of 24 lbs (11 kg). At first these results sound surprising. What had happened was that at the sixth week the hospitalized patients had been discharged and allowed to go home on an 800 calorie diet. The final weights of the two groups indicated that there was no great advantage in taking people into hospital, with all the trouble and expense that entailed. The weight losses as out-patients could be equally good.

This was a very important trial, the summation of all the work done over an eight-year period. As in other trials, the question of safety was all-important. Nitrogen balance was studied and it was shown that nitrogen losses were very small. Serum electrolytes were examined. Monthly electrocardiographs indicated no changes. The tests were remarkable in showing that the patients who used the diet were fit and well.

Our findings, to which A. Grant, O. Edwards and E.R. Littlewood also lent their names, were published in a refereed report in the December issue of *The International Journal of Obesity* in 1978. It was this paper which led directly to the launching of the Cambridge Diet in the United States in 1980, because it was read by Jack Feather, a wealthy Californian, who decided it was worth doing something positive about it. The story is told in Chapter 13.

CHAPTER TWELVE

AT THE CLINICS

Much of the work towards the end of the research period was carried out at Addenbrooke's Hospital in Cambridge, where an Obesity Clinic was specially set up for work on the Cambridge Diet. The first doctor in charge was Dr Ray Moore, a senior registrar whose particular interest was in the effects of weight reduction on metabolism. Within a few weeks, there were some 40 obese patients who came for treatment regularly. Since a senior registrar is rarely permanent, Ray Moore was followed by a succession of others and altogether some seven doctors have seen several hundred patients.

The treatment of obesity is not a popular subject among hospital doctors. Before the advent of the Cambridge Diet, overweight patients usually attended regular clinics and were then referred to the hospital dietician, who, more often than not, recommended a conventional 800-1000 calorie diet. They rarely lost weight and doctors were not specifically involved. However, with the new treatment, using the Cambridge Diet, an Obesity Clinic became very rewarding. Obese patients can be the most interesting of characters and it was extremely satisfying to see them succeeding for the first time in their lives, and to join in the enthusiasm their success created. The doctors often remarked that it was the most enjoyable clinic they held.

The Enthusiastic Physicians

In our endeavours we were joined by a number of other groups in Europe and in the United States. From all these clinics came enthusiastic reports from doctors that the weight losses were excellent and the diet in their hands appeared to be very safe.

Dr J. H. Paul Wilson, of Rotterdam, thought the new formula was a major advance in therapy for the massively obese patients who, on conventional diets, would need many years to achieve their ideal weight. Using the new formula he found that patients could lose between 3-4½ lbs (1.3–2 kg) a week consistently. Of the 90 patients he studied, a substantial number stayed on the diet for three or four months and some for as long as 11 months. They had an average weight loss of 22 lbs (10 kg) in four weeks and no serious side effects were seen. One woman started at 348 lbs (158 kg) and lost 187 lbs (85 kg) in 15 months, achieving her ideal weight of 150 lbs (68 kg), which he considered a remarkable achievement in view of previous failure on other diets.

Dr Noel Hickey, of Dublin, reported that on the basis of his own clinical trials the diet was a remarkable advance in medical treatment and quite different from crash diets extremely popular among the public. In his hands the new formula diet was extremely successful in producing very substantial weight reduction of the same order as that seen in complete starvation, without all the associated hazards. In Ireland, most doctors are loathe to put patients on conventional diets, because the drop-out rate is so high and it is usually a waste of time, because a year to two later they have regained all the weight. It is here that the new formulation scores. Because patients lose a great deal of weight rapidly, they are stimulated to change their eating habits so as to achieve permanent weight loss. At his clinic, he studied 14 people in which the average weight losses at four weeks were 17 lbs (7 kg) for men and 11½ lbs (5 kg) for women. At eight weeks the mean weight losses were 29 lbs (13 kg) for men and 18½ lbs (8 kg) for women. Such results are impossible to achieve using conventional diets. Although they were consuming only 330 calories, the patients lost their hunger after only a few days on the diet, a fact which I found very impressive.

The Critics

Not everyone in the scientific community approved of the Cambridge Diet. After its launch in the USA, and later in the UK, there began a flood of articles, notes and reviews criticizing the Cambridge Diet. Among the most vociferous were the leader writer of the Journal of the American Medical Association who claimed the diet was dangerous. To support their claim they drew attention to the small loss of lean body mass which occurs while on the diet. What the experts failed to appreciate is that there is no way in which any overweight individual could fail to lose lean body mass on any weight loss programme.

Lean body mass is defined as 'the total weight of the body minus its fatty tissue'. For instance, if you weigh 200 lbs (91 kg) and have 80 lbs (36 kg) of fatty tissue, your lean body mass is 120 lbs (55 kg). Basically it consists of the skeleton and the soft tissues of the body, particularly the muscles.

Using some very sophisticated measuring techniques, a very able British worker, Doctor Phillip James (now of the Rowett Research Institute, Bucksburn, Scotland), showed that overweight people had much more lean body mass than their lean counterparts. This is a logical finding, because if an individual has a lot of body fat to carry around, he will need a lot of muscle to support it. To give an example, if a man is 50 lbs (23 kg) overweight, about 36 per cent or 18 lbs (8 kg) of this excess weight is lean body mass. This is equivalent to about

4 lbs (2 kg) of protien, a quantity much larger than anyone ever anticipated and which provides a substantial store of this nutrient. If the 50 lbs (23 kg) over weight man goes on a diet and reaches his ideal weight, his body will receive an extra bonus of 4 lbs (2 kg) of protein to use for his nutritional needs. This loss of protein and lean body mass occurs on any diet whenever weight is lost, not just the Cambridge Diet.

In our original work on the development of the Cambridge Diet, we carefully measured the nitrogen losses occurring in patients while in hospital. It was found that over a four-week period, the difference between nitrogen intake and that excreted was only 55 grams. This is equivalent to about ¾ lb protein. From the weight loss which had occured could be calculated the amount of nitrogen excreted due to the loss of body protein, which must of necessity arise during weight loss. It was established that the nitrogen excreted was no greater than one would expect in a person losing that particular amount of weight.

One of the charges made by the JAMA experts was that if loss of lean body mass does occur it could come from the heart. Again, their criticism might apply to any weight loss diet. There is absolutely no evidence that there are changes to the heart muscle in patients receiving the Cambridge Diet. Studies have been conducted on hundreds of patients in metabolic wards and in out-patients clinics, in many centres in Europe and the United States and *no* heart changes associated with the Cambridge Diet have been seen. This even applies when studies were continued on patients using the Diet for up to four months as sole source. One of the techniques used by the cardiologists at three different centres was continuous twenty-four hour monitoring of heart rhythms using a tape recorder. No changes were seen in any significance while patients were on the Cambridge Diet.

None of the scientists who criticized the diet had ever

used it in their clinics. What really happened in both the United States and the United Kingdom speaks very much against their conclusions. Many general practitioners, after a few months, found that the Cambridge Diet was effective and very safe. They realized that with their limited time it was impossible to treat all the overweight patients in their practice individually. So they would hand them over to the nurse (who really didn't have any time for the patient, either). The solution was to bring in a well trained Cambridge Counsellor. Of course, if the patient was extremely overweight and wanted to go sole source for periods of several months, then the doctor would see that person regularly, but otherwise he would not need to spend his valuable time in this manner. A recent survey of general practitioners in the UK showed that 50% of them would recommend the diet to their patients.

It is estimated that over 5 million people used the Cambridge Diet in the USA and several hundred thousand in the UK. In this large number all investigations have proved to be minor. The predictions of the armchair critics that the Cambridge Diet is dangerous has not been seen in pratice.

Other Beneficial Effects

Many of the doctors who studied the Cambridge Diet were specialists in a wide number of medical subjects, such as nutrition, endocrinology, diabetes and cardiovascular disease. Besides weight loss, they were also interested in the subsidiary beneficial effects of the Diet, several of which came to light. Much of this was reported at the two scientific conferences on the Cambridge Diet, one held on the island of Ischia, near Naples, in October 1980, and the other in Falmouth, Cape Cod, Massachusetts, in June 1983.

Diabetes

The risk of developing diabetes is very high in over-weight people. In fact, the majority of people who become diabetic when adults are overweight, and most doctors, on examining a diabetic for the first time, will recommend weight loss as an important part of their treatment. Diabetics, like most other overweight people, find it extremely difficult to lose weight and maintain their weight loss on conventional diets. With an introduction of the Cambridge Diet their lives have been made much easier, because they can also succeed. One of the doctors who has a particular interest in diabetes is Mario Mancini of the Polyclinic in Naples. He took a number of overweight mild diabetics and put them on the Cambridge Diet as their sole form of treatment for six weeks. After a few days, their blood sugar became normal and their high blood fats (cholesterol and trigly-cerides) also decreased. These beneficial changes continued until the end of their treatment.

Other doctors have found that when treating diabetics with the Cambridge Diet, it is necessary to reduce patients' medication. Among these is Dr Jerrold Olesky of the University of San Diego, who is currently examining a large group of overweight diabetics. He, like many others, was very impressed with the ease with which they lost weight. He feels that the Cambridge Diet is a valuable tool for the study of diabetes. For the first time it is possible to reduce the weight of large numbers of patients and to study the contribution which obesity makes towards the disease.

Blood Fats

The treatment of high blood fats has been of special interest to me and Dr Ian McLean Baird for many years. It was therefore very encouraging for us to find that the Cambridge Diet reduced blood cholesterol by 25 per cent and triglycerides by 40 per cent. Every single patient who undergoes the Cambridge Diet for weight loss shows a decrease in blood fat, especially those who had high levels to start with. Most of these people, who were at high risk for coronary heart disease, were able to get their blood fats down to normal by using the diet. However, this was only achieved while they were using the diet sole source. On returning to a normal diet their blood fats increased again, although not to such high levels as were seen previously.

High Blood Pressure

It is very common for the overweight person to suffer from high blood pressure. A drop in blood pressure is seen within a few days of starting the diet, even when weight loss is still quite small. On achievement of normal weight, blood pressure is often brought down completely to normal.

To give an example, one patient, Robert Walton of Little Paxton reported the following: 'My wife works for a doctor, and one day he asked several of us if he could try out his new blood pressure machine, using us as patients. I was most happy to oblige as I was quite sure I had no problems with my blood pressure. You can imagine my surprise, and the doctor's concern, when my blood pressure registered 200/130! As I am only 36 years of age, it didn't seem possible. In fact, he even took it again, and when it remained the same we all thought there might be something wrong with the machine. As it turned out, the machine was correct.

'At about this time [early May 1984] friends introduced me to the Cambridge Diet. My weight was 14st 3 (199 lbs; 90 kg). I went on the diet as my sole source of nutrition for one month and by 30th May my blood pressure registered 150/105! I had a one-week maintenance period and then went back sole source for another week. By 6th June my blood pressure was 145/93 and kept going down until 29th June when it reached 125/90. I had lost the weight I had been trying to get off and then weighed 12 st. 10 (169 lbs; 76 kg). A loss of 30 lbs (13 kg).

'By taking the Cambridge Diet for weight maintenance and for nutrition, I have easily been able to keep my blood pressure at a normal range. The doctor has been quite amazed at my progress and fully encourages me to stay with the Cambridge Diet formula as a means of controlling my blood pressure.'

Two doctors who have made the subject of special interest are Dr Dvornik of Washington State and Dr Stephen Kreitzman, Emory University, Atlanta, Georgia. Their studies on the effect of the Cambridge Diet on high blood pressure are still continuing and are likely to prove of great interest to the medical profession in the future.

The standard treatment of high blood pressure is to give medication. Unfortunately the drugs do not cure the condition and therefore have to be taken for very long periods, often for life. Throughout the world there are millions of people affected and the total cost of medication is enormous. If weight reduction, using the Cambridge Diet, could cause a permanent decrease in blood pressure in even a proportion of those affected, there would be a great saving in both time and money.

Thyroid Hormones

As mentioned in Chapter 1, people who lose weight usually decrease their metabolism after a week or two and those on the Cambridge Diet are no exception. After four weeks there is a 20 per cent drop in the basal metabolic rate, which can lead to a fall in the rate of weight loss. Many patients who have been on the diet for 12 to 16 weeks find that their weight loss slows to about half of what it was at the beginning. This decrease in metabolism is due to a fall in blood thyroid hormone levels and the sites on cells at which the hormone acts. The subject has received special study by Drs Paul Wilson and Steve Lamberts of Rotterdam and Dr Ray Moore in Cambridge.

To understand the subject further it is necessary to delve into the question of thyroid hormones. The thyroid gland makes a hormone called T4 (with four iodine atoms in the molecule) which is converted in the tissues into T3 (with three iodine atoms) — the active form of the hormone. It has been found that people following the Cambridge Diet for several weeks, have a decreased level of T3 in their blood plasma. Dr Ray Moore hit upon the idea of restoring the deficiency of T3 by giving small doses of this hormone (about 20 micro grams) three times a day. He took two groups of patients, all of whom had reached a plateau in their weight loss after 12 weeks; to one group he gave T3 and to the other he gave a dummy tablet. The group given T3 showed a marked improvement in their rate of weight loss and the level of T3 in their plasma became normal. The other untreated group were unchanged and their weight loss was still very slow.

The results, published in the *Lancet*, were of great interest to doctors and many of them now use T3 as a supplementary treatment to the Cambridge Diet when required. It is quite common at our Obesity Clinic at Addenbrooke's Hospital for the doctor to prescribe small doses of T3 to patients who plateau, and more often than not they feel the benefit by once again continuing their weight loss.

Anti-Depressants

One of the problems of slimming diets is that patients often become depressed. This has not been a complication of the Cambridge Diet; in fact, the reverse is true. Usually people report that they have never felt happier in the whole of their lives. One of the senior registrars, Dr Russell Cook of Addenbrooke's Hospital, had a special interest in depression and decided to investigate this aspect using some sophisticated questionnaires which he had devised.

For his study, he used the anti-depressant drug, Miaserin. Half the patients were treated with the drug and the remainder with a dummy tablet. Altogether thirty patients were given the Cambridge Diet sole source for sixteen weeks. He found that most patients on the Cambridge Diet were not depressed at all and that Miaserin made no difference to their state of mind, or weight loss. Although the study was negative from his point of view, in that the drug had no beneficial effect, the information he obtained coincidentally about the diet was most helpful. From a variety of biochemical and clinical tests, he found that the thirty patients were healthy and well at the end of the sixteen weeks. It was his work that gave us great confidence to treat large number of patients at the obesity clinic for long periods of time, often six to nine months, knowing that the treatment was safe. In fact, it is as safe from six to nine months as it is at four to eight weeks.

Multiple Sclerosis

Through the Counsellor system in the United States, we began to hear some interesting reports about a number of overweight people who also had multiple sclerosis. Many of these MS sufferers said that their symptoms were improved after using the diet and that they went into remission. Carolyn Petersen, a young wife and mother, had been diagnosed MS for several years, and before she went on to the diet she was unable to walk without help. Her speech was impaired, her vision was bad and she was unable to feel anything with her hands and feet. After six months of using the Cambridge Diet, mostly sole source, she lost all her excess weight and during the process most of her symptoms disappeared. Suddenly she found that not only could she walk, she could run! Her speech came back completely, as did her ability to feel objects.

Many patients with MS show a spontaneous remission of their symptoms. Yet it is impossible, using only a few examples, to show that any benefit can be attributed directly to the diet. Therefore, together with Eleanor Harnish (whose story is given in Chapter 5), I decided to carry out a pilot study giving the Cambridge Diet to about twenty-five MS patients. The trial is still continuing. The results so far have been encouraging, in that the condition of most people has improved slightly. However there is no evidence that the Cambridge Diet cures the disease.

It will take many years before it is known whether or not the current line of research will be of any significance, but as the cause of multiple sclerosis is still unknown, it is important to follow up any new lead whenever it arises.

Future Research in Obesity

Much more research into the cause of obesity is needed at the present time. Of course, everyone knows that people become overweight because they eat more than they need. Yet many thin people exist who have very healthy appetites and consume large amounts of food without getting fat. Research studies have shown that the intake of food of fat people is usually no greater than that consumed by thin people, but the metabolism of fat people may be lower.

Obese people are something of a paradox, because their resting metabolic rate is actually higher than that of thin people. However, the total daily energy expenditure of fat people must be considerably lower otherwise they would not remain fat. The major question is: how do thin people expend more energy? Is it through more physical activity or during the digestion of food? Current research in several laboratories throughout the world suggests that, when a person eats, much of the energy is expended in the digestive process. In other words, the thin person 'burns off' much of the energy he consumes and releases it as heat.

It is in this area of research that the Cambridge Diet can be of most value, by providing a research tool for converting fat people into thin people. When someone becomes fat, measurements made on them are often the result of their being fat and may not reflect any abnormality they possess. By taking fat people and slimming them down to normal weight, it is possible to study 'fat people' who are at the same weight as their thin counterparts. Studies made of such people are likely to be more valuable in finding out why some of us are fat and others thin. Before the advent of the Cambridge Diet it was difficult to do such investigations, because there was no diet which could guarantee weight loss in sufficient numbers to make such experiments worthwhile.

It is this line of research that my group in Cambridge is now actively pursuing.

CHAPTER THIRTEEN

THE FINANCIAL HURDLES

Research is expensive. It requires facilities, salaried technical staff and money to pay for chemicals and routine analyses. Before embarking on new projects, every scientist has to ensure that suitable funds are available. In 1970, when work on the diet started, research support from government sources, such as the Medical Research Council, was severely curtailed. Those of us engaged in the research relied chiefly on pharmaceutical companies, which were often willing to invest in a project which might be of commercial interest to them.

In January 1970, the medical weekly, the *Lancet*, carried an advertisement from a company named Vivonex, asking if anyone was interested in research on their product. On further inquiry, I discovered that Vivonex was a complete diet of 2,000 calories, which had been developed for astronauts undertaking space missions. The idea was to produce a completely synthetic food substitute, composed of a mixture of amino-acids, which left little or no residue, so that stools from astronauts could be kept to a minimum. Unfortunately, astronauts preferred real food and were not satisfied with the unpalatable mixture Vivonex had prepared. Nevertheless, I saw that it might be possible to modify the Vivonex formula into the perfect slimming diet. I contacted the company in California and they agreed, through their London representative, to supply research funds. Materials were flown over from

Mountain View, California, to London so that the work could begin.

The project had been under way for only a few months, when we learned that the Vivonex Corporation had been taken over by Eaton Laboratories, a subsidiary of Morton-Norwich, a large American company which originally made its profits from selling salt. A meeting was arranged with Eaton Laboratories at their London office. The new owners of Vivonex acknowledged that our work was important and interesting, and agreed to continue supporting it.

By the end of 1971, the first trial with the Vivonex mixture was completed, and the results were astonishing. It was possible, it seemed, for fat people to live on as little as 250 calories per day. My patent agent assured me that the diet was an original concept and I decided to register a provisional patent application in the United Kingdom in March 1972.

The next twelve months saw very active discussions with the Board of Morton-Norwich, to ascertain their interest and, as a result, a satisfactory licence agreement was worked out. One year later, patent applications were applied for in twelve other countries, including the United States. The Board of Morton-Norwich decided to meet the patent costs and to provide finance for staff salaries and all outgoing expenses. To clinch the deal, I flew out to Norwich, New York, calling at Philadelphia on the way to pick up my United States lawyer and patent agent. The latter turned out to be an amateur pilot and I still have sleepless nights remembering that single-engine prop-plane trip from Philadelphia to Norwich, New York!

Everything went well for a time, and then to our dismay, the Board of Morton-Norwich replaced their President with someone who did not look favourably on our research. The Morton-Norwich decision to drop our project seemed catastrophic at the time. Trials with the egg albumin diet had been successful and everything seemed to be going according to plan. Suddenly I had to look for somebody else to support the work.

I wrote to all the major food companies in the United States, Canada and Europe, among them Beechams and Glaxo in Britain, and the Swiss giant, Hoffmann-La Roche. I had previously had personal contact with many of their senior management or research staff and informed them that initial trials had been a great success and that there were patents to cover the product.

After innumerable meetings in many different cities around the world, the negative answers came in with monotonous regularity. Everyone said that the diet had great potential and was just what the public needed. Yet somewhere between those to whom I spoke and the management that made decisions was a block which I could not penetrate. It was a difficult period, but we were fortunate enough to have some funds left over to carry on for a short time.

Eventually good fortune came our way through the agency of Dennis Jones, an old student of mine who became a junior lecturer at the Department of Applied Biology at Cambridge and later joined the large multi-national company, Organon, which had its headquarters in the town of Oss, in central Holland. Through his introduction, I became an adviser to Organon after visiting their research group and giving a lecture about my work on coronary heart disease. At the appropriate time, I put the idea to Dennis Jones that the management of Organon might be interested in supporting our pioneer work on dieting. Dennis Jones worked well behind the scenes and eventually convinced Organon of the worthiness of the project. There then followed a very happy collaboration with the people at Organon, who over the next three years spent more than £100,000 in developing the new diet, with Dennis Jones as the project leader.

The Howard Diet

The first step in making the new diet was to find a factory capable of manufacturing the basic diet material to my specifications. The company chosen belonged to one of our largest food groups, Lyons-Tetley at Market Harborough, about 50 miles from Cambridge, where technical staff had become experts in devising soups and milk shakes. My formula then employing milk as a protein source, was converted into chicken and asparagus soups, as well as banana, raspberry, peach and strawberry milk shakes. These flavours were a great improvement on what had been developed before and received a tolerant, if unenthusiastic, response from patients.

The so-called 'Howard Diet' was then tested in a number of centres, principally Addenbrooke's Hospital in Cambridge and the West Middlesex Hospital in Isleworth, just as if it had been a new drug. Each patient was seen weekly, and frequent samples of blood were taken for biochemical analysis. After a study of several hundred patients, using a battery of routine tests, including electrocardiographs and other clinical examinations, the diet was found remarkably effective, and absolutely no adverse effects of any importance were discovered.

Yet Organon did not wish to rely solely on the results from the two obesity clinics, and enrolled six other clinics in different parts of Europe to evaluate the Howard Diet. Organon had good contacts with Dr Paul Wilson and Dr Steven Lamberts at the Department of Internal Medicine at the University of Rotterdam, and also with Dr Noel Hickey, Dr Geoffrey Bourke and Dr Risteard Mulcahy at University Hospital, Dublin. At this time, I was already giving lectures throughout Europe on the new diet and had been particularly well received in Copenhagen, Gothenburg and Naples. All these groups decided to take part in formal trials. In addition, Dr Harold Shapiro in Manchester, a general practitioner with a large obesity practice, decided to compare the Howard Diet with his standard 600 calorie food diet. Altogether, eight centres were involved in the final testing. Without exception they agreed that the diet was extremely effective and quite safe.

Randolph de Bruin, head of the Clinical Department at Organon, produced an enthusiastic report. He had been especially interested in the trials at Rotterdam, because of his personal associations with Dr Paul Wilson. However, not everyone supported it. Organon had also conducted palatability trials in France and reported that the general acceptance of the taste was not encouraging and that he was sceptical whether ordinary members of the public would take to the diet. He was no doubt right to pronounce the diet poor in taste; nevertheless the drop-out rate in all the trials had been extremely low, much lower than with ordinary diets. We countered his argument with our view that people on slimming diets seldom expect to be treated with the flavour of gourmet food. For six months there was silence while the Organon Board deliberated.

Competitors

About the same time as our collaboration with Morton-Norwich, two American scientists had also hit on the idea of developing a new, very low calorie treatment for massively obese diabetics. They were Saul Genuth and Victor Vertes of Cleveland, Ohio. Both our groups met at the First International Congress on Obesity in London in 1973 to present our results to the world for the first time.

Genuth and Vertes were being supported financially by the Delmark Company of the U.S.A. The latter was controlled by the Swiss giant pharmaceutical company, Sandoz, which also included Wander as one of its Swiss subsidiaries. Their formulation was based on egg albumin as the source of protein. It was eventually sold in the United States as Optifast and in Europe as Modifast.

Genuth and Vertes insisted that the diet should only be used by skilled physicians who specialized in the treatment of the overweight in special clinics. Altogether they liaised with doctors on the treatment of hundreds of patients throughout the United States. Their trials were very successful and like ourselves, they saw few side effects.

While all this was happening in the U.S.A., Sandoz had its eyes on Europe, and particularly Germany, which is their biggest market. Getting wind of the Organon trials, they decided to speed up their marketing plans in Europe, and in the summer of 1978 introduced Modifast to pharmacies in Germany and Holland. Organon were well and truly beaten to the post. I believe that the Howard Diet was more palatable than Modifast. It was certainly cheaper and if it could have been launched it would have competed well.

Wander found their product was a moderate commercial success on the continent. Subsequently, they introduced it in the United Kingdom in 1980, where it became available from pharmacies with the recommendation of general practitioners, who had been circularized with a great deal of literature about it.

Another country in which there was activity was Denmark. In 1978, I visited the University of Copenhagen to give a lecture at the Hvidovre Hospital to Professor Fleming Quaade and his group. He is the most respected expert in the treatment of obesity in Denmark and his prime interest at that time was in surgical operations. Together with a colleague he had developed an improved method for stomach stapling.

After my lecture on the Howard Diet, he was extremely impressed with the results obtained and felt that there might now be no need for these operations. He therefore decided to carry out a comparative study, using the Howard Diet on one or two of his patients. Although he was impressed with their weight loss, which was equivalent to that obtained with his operations, he did not like the flavours and subsequently decided to devise his own formulation based on orange juice and soya protein. Since he was a little uncertain of the exact formulation, he asked my advice. I flew to Copenhagen and met him and his colleague, Oluf Mork, and was delighted when they agreed to formulate a new diet of almost exactly the same composition as the Howard Diet, because it would independently confirm my results. An endorsement of the safety of my diet was of greater value than any commercial considerations. Their clinical trials were very successful and Professor Quaade was able to confirm the safety of the Howard Diet in his own clinic. Oluf Mork now distributes in Denmark a composition under the name 'Nupo', which is available in several flavours and is sold in health food stores and supermarkets.

Because of its greater palatability and more effective method of distribution, it was decided to introduce the Cambridge Diet in Denmark in the spring of 1985 under the name Cambridge Kuren, where it is made available through the Cambridge Counsellor system.

The Feathers

After many months of waiting, Organon management summoned me to Oss to tell me personally that they had reluctantly decided not to proceed with the marketing of the Howard Diet. Clearly the appearance of Modifast in Germany and The Netherlands was the deciding factor and Organon accepted defeat. I was to be persuaded to assign the patent rights to Sandoz for whatever sum Organon could get. This was entirely unacceptable. Having spent years developing our diet, the last thing I wished to see was all the work dissipated for the sake of a rival product. Clearly the Organon management wanted to recoup some of their large investment. Eventually talks broke down and Organon gave up any claim they had to the patent rights, and yet again we had to look for another sponsor.

It was not too long before further support was found. In the summer of 1979, Jack and Eileen Feather, two Californian multi-millionaires, decided to put a considerable part of their fortune into a new venture. They chose to support the Howard Diet (which then became known as the Cambridge Diet).

Jack and Eileen grew up in the mid-west in upper-middle-class homes and as a newly married couple emigrated to California, where Jack enrolled at the University of California to study literature. Within six months of entering the course he came down with a serious case of polio and the doctors thought he was crippled for life, a decision the couple refused to accept. Over the years he had developed an intense interest in nutrition and exercise which he then applied to his medical condition. The results were quite dramatic. Within eighteen months he had made a remarkable recovery that amazed all his doctors. The secret of Jack's success was the use of what he called 'negative exercise'. In no time, the news spread, and Jack was asked to help others with similar problems. As a result he rented an 800 sq. ft (74 sq. m.) store and converted it into a health club in Berkeley. Besides helping medical cases, many of their clientele were people who just wanted to improve their looks or their body shape. The business grew and grew and they established many other health clubs. This involved a great deal of hard work for both Jack and Eileen. As a result they became extremely wealthy.

Jack had always been interested in nutritional research, and in 1975 he set about producing a new and revolutionary slimming diet. After three-and-a-half years of

144

work, he and his son, Vaughn, had been able to develop a product which they felt ready to market. Before doing so, the Feathers decided to take a short vacation to their summer home in England. Jack took with him on the plane a stack of scientific journals to read, including some back issues of the *International Journal of Obesity*. By the time dinner was being served, Jack had reached the 1978 December issue of the journal and our article about the Howard Diet.

Jack was quite amazed by what he read, because it was very close to the ideas which he and his son had worked on, but better. This English mansion in Surrey was quite close to the West Middlesex Hospital, and in no time at all they contacted Dr Ian McLean Baird and arranged a meeting. When they heard that the product was covered by a United States patent they were extremely excited and anxious to obtain the rights.

An agreement was quickly reached and the Feathers began their marketing of our diet by mail order in March of the following year. This was followed early in 1981 by the Counsellor system and direct sales. It was they who chose to change the name of the 'Howard Diet' to the Cambridge Diet, and their new company was called Cambridge Plan International.

The Feathers had in their hands a remarkable diet which had been developed at no cost to themselves. All the money for its development had been paid for by Morton-Norwich and Organon. It was endorsed by a galaxy of International medical experts and emanated from one of the world's prestigious universities.

Through their efforts, the system of marketing by Cambridge Counsellors was evolved; a method of distribution that was so much more beneficial than selling cans of diet through chemists.

In their own development they had achieved considerable expertise in flavouring. The new Cambridge Diet was a huge leap ahead in palatability compared with the old Howard Diet. Overweight Americans liked the flavours and the diet became extremely successful.

The success of the Cambridge Diet can be measured by the number of companies which attempted to rival the formulation. Altogether, there were more than fifty. Their products were sold under the name 'Oxford Diet', 'Eton Diet', 'University Diet', and many other names, and were chiefly retailed from chemists' shops. Patent infringement actions were vigorously pursued in the courts. In South Africa, a Johannesburg entrepreneur cheekily introduced his 'NEW' Cambridge Diet, while in the United Kingdom, Univite 330, a close copy of the Cambridge Diet, was made available in 1983 by mail order and later through the counsellor-type system as 'The Micro Diet'. None of these is exactly formulated according to the results of stringent tests which produced the original 'Cambridge Diet'.

In retrospect, the decisions of Morton-Norwich and Organon to drop the diet were a blessing in disguise. The Feather family, in deciding to take up the Cambridge Diet made a significant contribution to medical science and the treatment of obesity in particular.

My involvement with Cambridge Plan International has been very limited. Although I was occasionally invited to give a lecture or was asked for advise on medical and scientific matters, the business organization was completely outside my sphere of influence. The situation in Britain is different. I have wanted the Diet to be available in Britain for many years but for one reason or another the plans were continually postponed.

In April 1984, a decision was taken to start a new company in Britain called Cambridge Nutrition Ltd., completely independent of the Feather family.

The U.K. company is wholly owned by a British charity, The Howard Foundation, whose objects are to assist bio-medical research in obesity, coronary heart disease, diabetes, multiple sclerosis and Third World nutrition. The company is headed by my brother, Dr Roger Howard, a biochemist who returned from the United States to take on the challenge of making the Diet available to the many millions of obesity sufferers in this country.

The patent rights for the Cambridge Diet are owned by a charity called 'The William Harvey Foundation', which receives royalties from the Cambridge Diet and uses the money for the benefit of biomedical research and education. A substantial part of these royalties are donated to the Howard Foundation and the trustees, of which I am one, have a special interest in Third World Nutrition. One of the projects currently being supported by the foundation is the publication of a new journal called *Hunger*. This will be a politically independent periodical in which people can explain their views freely and suggest how the problem of feeding the undernourished in the Third World can best be solved.

PART III

A Compendium of Useful Information

CHAPTER FOURTEEN

NUTRITIONAL INFORMATION

A Complete Diet

A complete diet by definition contains every substance the body needs for perfect health. The body needs *energy* which is provided by carbohydrates, alcohol, fat and protein. It requires protein for the *repair* of body tissues. Minerals, trace elements, vitamins and fibre are needed for its proper *structure and function*.

Recommended Daily Allowance (RDA)

To meet the known nutritional needs of the average healthy person, levels of intake of essential nutrients have been calculated which, on the basis of current knowledge, are considered to be adequate. Although many committees have suggested figures, those provided by the Food and Nutrition Board in the United States are the most comprehensive and complete. For brevity, the term RDA (for Recommended Daily Allowance) will be frequently used in what follows here. The figures given in Table 1 (page 152) are for adults and are based on American recommendations. Where men and woman differ, the higher figure is quoted.

Energy

Energy is most often measured in calories. A calorie is defined as the amount of heat required to raise the

TABLE I RECOMMENDED DAILY ALLOWANCES (USA)

Protein	men 56g women 46g		
Fat	1-2% calorie intake		
Fibre	30g*		

Vitamins	mg	*Minerals and Trace Elements*	mg
A	1	Calcium	800
B$_1$	1.5	Phosphorus	800
B$_2$	1.7	Magnesium	350
Niacin	18	Potassium	1900*
B$_6$	0.1	Chloride	1700
Pantothenic Acid	0.1*	Iron	18
Biotin	0.2*	Zinc	15
Folic Acid	0.4	Iodine	0.15
B$_{12}$	0.003	Copper	2*
C	60	Manganese	2.5*
D	0.01	Selenium	0.05*
E	10	Molybdenum	0.15*
K	0.14	Chromium	0.05*

* There is no offical RDA, but figures quoted are considered
adequate

temperature of 1cc water one degree centigrade. In scientific textbooks the energy content of most foods is given in kilocalories (1000 calories), but non-scientists usually drop the prefix 'kilo'. To avoid confusion, I have done so throughout this book. Some people prefer to measure energy in joules. One joule is equivalent to 0.238 Kcal.

Table 2 gives the caloric contents (per gram) of the different food types.

The body has reserves of energy. The amount of carbohydrate is extremely limited and in complete starvation is used up in 1-2 days. For its long-term energy

TABLE 2 CALORIES/G (KCAL/G)

Protein	4
Carbohydrate	4
Fat	9
Alcohol	7
Vitamins, Minerals	0
Trace elements	0
Fibre	0

needs, the body has to burn up fat, and in certain circumstances (such as in complete starvation) protein.

Protein

Protein is made up from 'building bricks' known as amino-acids. Altogether there are twenty-two, of which eight are essential. These are: Isoleucine, Leucine, Lysine, Methionine, Phenylalanine, Threonine, Tryptophan and Valine. If the diet does not contain enough of the 'essential' amino-acids, protein cannot be made in the body and its tissue eventually wastes away. Proteins provide the basic structural compounds of living cells. They are mostly found in the muscle tissue and the remainder in soft tissues such as liver, kidney and lung and also in teeth, blood and other fluids.

Protein is being continually made and destroyed. If the diet does not contain adequate protein, severe damage will occur to vital organs such as the heart.

The RDA for protein is 56g for men and 46g for women. The Cambridge Diet contains only 33 grams of protein, which is less than the RDA. This is because in our investigations it was found that obese people receiving only 330 calories do not require such a large quantity of protein (see Chapter 11 for explanation).

Fat

Although the body contains a lot of fat (and in over-weight people, too much), the amount of fat needed in the diet is very small, being just a few grams of essential fatty acids (EFA). The chief of these is linoleic acid. A deficiency of EFA is difficult to produce in man but in other animals a skin rash and anaemia is seen. EFA is important for the production of the prostaglandins, which are important substances in the body which regulate blood pressure, heart rate and the function of nerves.

Much of the fat we eat is non-essential and consists of saturated fatty acids, a high intake of which raises the cholesterol content of the blood and is a risk factor for coronary heart disease.

Carbohydrate

Besides fat, carbohydrate is the main source of energy in our diet. It is stored in the liver and muscles as glycogen for short-term energy requirements. Carbohydrates, or chemicals derived from them, are important constituents of cells, connective tissue and nerves, and in the liver they remove toxic products. When the carbohydrate in the diet is low (or absent), fat cannot be burned up completely and substances called 'ketones' are formed. These can be used by the brain instead of glucose. When ketones accumulate in the blood, 'ketosis' is said to develop. A mild 'ketosis' is not harmful and people may experience a feeling of 'euphoria' (or happiness). Since muscle protein can be broken down and converted into carbohydrates, a deficiency never occurs and there is no RDA. Carbohydrates also retain electrolytes in the body.

Vitamins

Vitamins are a group of chemical compounds which are needed in only minute quantity and which are essential for the proper functioning of the body.

Vitamin A Also known as retinol – an essential component of the retina of the eye, and important in bone and skin growth. A deficiency causes 'night blindness'. High levels of vitamin A are toxic.

Vitamin B-1 Known also as thiamine, this is an essential part of an enzyme system necessary for the breakdown of carbohydrate. B-1 deficiency causes a disease called 'beri-beri', which is characterized by weakness, numbness in the legs, and paralysis.

Vitamin B-2 Also known as riboflavin, this vitamin is also extremely important in key enzyme systems in the breakdown of carbohydrates and fat. A deficiency is characterized by cracks in the skin, and eye disease.

Niacin (or Nicotinamide) An important component of several enzyme systems and necessary for the breakdown of fat and carbohydrate. A deficiency leads to the disease 'pellagra', characterized by weakness, fatigue, and ulceration of the mouth and tongue.

Vitamin B-6 Also known as pyridoxine, and needed in many enzyme systems, particularly those involved in the breakdown of protein. A deficiency leads to skin disease and anaemia.

Pantothenic Acid An essential part of an important enzyme system, this functions in the synthesis and breakdown of carbohydrates, proteins and fats. Experimental deficiency in man produces a wide

155

variety of symptoms, particularly depression, fainting, rapid pulse and susceptibility to infection.

Biotin An important component of enzyme systems, involving the breakdown of fats and amino-acids. The deficiency is difficult to produce in man and animals. The chief abnormality is skin disease.

Folic Acid Involved in the formation of DNA and RNA, important constituents of all cells. A deficiency causes a special type of anaemia, in which the red cells are immature.

Vitamin B-12 Also called cyanocobalamin, this is essential for all cells, especially those of the gastro-intestinal tract, bone marrow and nervous tissue. As with folic acid, a deficiency of B-12 leads to anaemia caused by immaturity of the red cells. In addition, the function of the nervous system is affected.

Vitamin C Also known as ascorbic acid, this is needed for the normal function of cells. It is especially important in the adrenal gland, and the production and maintenance of collagen, a substance found in all fibrous tissue. It is abundant in the white cells of the blood, and thought to be important in the prevention of infection. A deficiency of Vitamin C leads to scurvy, which is characterized by skin haemorrhages, bleeding gums, and pains in the joints.

Vitamin D Another name for this is cholecaliferol. It is essential for the formation of bones and teeth and influences the absorption and use of calcium and phosphorus. A deficiency causes rickets in children, in which normal bone is not formed, and osteoporosis, a rarefaction of the bones in the elderly. Vitamin

D can be made in the body by the action of sunlight on the skin. In large doses it is toxic.

Vitamin E Also called tocopherol, of which a number of forms exist (alpha-tocopherol is the most important). It is a strong anti-oxidant and prevents the oxidation of unsaturated fatty acids, especially essential fatty acids. In deficiency states, there is an increased tendency for the red cells to become unstable and break up. Nowadays, the vitamin is synthesized as alpha-tocopherol acetate.

In some varieties of the Cambridge Diet (for instance in the United Kingdom), extra vitamin E is added as an anti-oxidant, to prevent the small quantity of fat going rancid.

Vitamin K Also known as menadione, this is required for the normal production of an enzyme in the blood called prothrombin, essential for blood clotting. A deficiency leads to an increased tendency to bleed, and haemorrhage; this is very unlikely to happen because bacteria make the vitamin in the intestine. In large amounts it is toxic.

Minerals

These are elements which are required by the body in relatively large amounts, and which are important in its structure and function.

Calcium The most abundant mineral in the body, since it is a major component, together with phosphorus, in the skeleton. It is also an important constituent of body fluids, especially the blood, where it is used in a large number of biochemical processes, such as blood clotting, nerve transmission, and regulation of the heart beat. A deficiency results in a tendency to develop rickets and osteomalacia. Together with vitamin D, it is all-important in preventing these.

Phosphorus Especially associated with calcium in the skeleton and in the body fluids. It is extremely important in many biochemical processes and is especially involved in the formation of DNA, RNA and phospholipids, which are key components of all cells. Like calcium, phosphorus is needed for the formation of healthy bones. An important point is that the ratio of calcium to phosphorus in the diet should be 1:1.

Magnesium An important constituent of bone, magnesium is a major constituent of fluid outside cells, and activates many enzymes. Magnesium deficiency can result in tetany (convulsions, cramps and muscle twitching), muscular weakness, and vertigo.

Potassium Most of the body's potassium is found inside the cells of the body, especially in muscle. It functions in regulating pH and the osmotic pressure of cells. It is necessary for the breakdown of carbohydrates and protein. A dietary deficiency can cause abnormal rhythm of the heart beats, and death from heart failure. Diuretics used for the treatment of high blood pressure often cause the elimination of potassium in the urine, and when potassium intake is low or restricted, the normal functioning of the heart may be adversely affected.

Sodium Surprisingly, about 30-45 per cent of the body's sodium is present in bone. It is a major component of the fluid surrounding cells and regulates pH, the osmotic pressure, and the amount of fluid in the body. It is difficult, if not impossible, to produce a dietary deficiency, since the body responds to lack by reducing its excretion. However, after a long period without sodium, a normal intake can lead to oedema – an accumulation of water in the joints. A high intake of sodium has been implicated in causing high blood pressure. There is no RDA of sodium but a moderately low intake is 1.5g, a low intake is less than 0.75g.

Chloride A component of the fluid surrounding cells, this activates enzymes, is involved in the maintenance of osmotic pressure, and is necessary for the breakdown of carbohydrates and protein. It is important in digestion, being part of the hydrochloric acid in the stomach. A deficiency can only occur when the body loses large amounts, as in vomiting, diarrhoea or sweating.

Sulphur The bulk of the sulphur in the body is in the sulphur-containing amino-acids. Although it is needed for metabolism, a deficiency of sulphur never occurs.

Trace Elements

These are required by the body in very small amounts, and are important in its structure and function, particularly the latter.

Iron Most iron is found in the red cells as haemoglobin but it is important in the transfer of oxygen and in several enzyme systems. A deficiency leads to anaemia.

Zinc Present in most tissues, including muscle and bone, zinc is an important constituent of insulin and many enzymes, including those affecting immunity. A deficiency in man produces anaemia, poor growth,

159

loss of hair, skin disease and a deficiency of male hormones.

Iodine This element is a constituent of the thyroid hormone synthesized in the thyroid gland, which controls the release of total energy in the body. A deficiency of iodine leads to goitre in which the thyroid gland enlarges.

Copper Found in the body tissues including liver, brain, heart and kidney, copper is involved in several enzyme systems. There is no evidence that copper deficiency can occur in man.

Manganese This is found in bone and several of the body tissues, and is important in enzyme systems, especially the liver. A deficiency has never been seen.

Fluorine Present in bone, fluorine reduces dental caries. Otherwise its nutritional importance is obscure. There is no RDA. Sufficient is now added to most drinking water or special toothpastes.

Selenium An important component of an enzyme acting as an anti-oxidant. It functions in concert with vitamin E to protect the cells against hydrogen peroxide formation.

Molybdenum This element is important in at least two enzyme processes.

Cobalt The important constituent of vitamin B-12. Enough cobalt is provided if there is sufficient B-12 in the diet.

Chromium The function of this element is obscure but it appears to be involved in the breakdown of glucose. A deficiency produces diabetes.

Fibre This is material which is undigested by the body and which is for the most part excreted. Nutritionists now believe that it is much more important than hitherto recognized in the prevention of intestinal disease, and possibly in preventing many others.

An Adequate and Balanced Diet

The success of planning nutritious meals centres on the inclusion of all the important nutrients in the amounts they are required, together with adequate calories. A good diet should contain all the RDAs of the nutrients discussed above. As a start, it is a good idea to know what foods contain each nutrient. Comprehensive food tables exist but they are very detailed and complex. The following list gives a brief guide to the sources of the major nutrients.

Protein Provided through meat, fish, poultry, eggs, milk and products made from milk, such as cheese. Vegetable proteins are contained in nuts, peas, beans and cereals.

Carbohydrate Cereals, fruit, vegetables such as potatoes, rice and pasta, all provide carbohydrate.

Fat Fat is found in meat, egg and cheese, butter, margarine, cream and oils.

Vitamins, Minerals and Trace Elements These are provided by most natural food. Some foods contain more than others, for example fruit and vegetables contain vitamin C, which is only in small quantities or absent in other foods.

Fibre Contained in whole wheat, fruit and vegetables, especially peas and beans.

The Four Food Groups Variety of food is important to obtain a wide range of nutrients. Some foods make major contributions. For example, milk is an important source of calcium, phosphorus and riboflavin. Table 3 (see below) gives a foundation for a good diet based on four food groups: meat, milk, vegetables/fruit and cereals. By choosing a wide variety of foods from each group it is possible to obtain adequate nutrition containing all the RDAs.

TABLE 3 FOUNDATION OF AN ADEQUATE DIET

Type of Food Group	Minimum Serving Recommended/Day	Servings
Meat	2	Lean meat, poultry or fish (2-3 oz; 56-85g) 2 eggs
Milk	2	milk (8oz; 227 ml whole or skimmed) cheese (1⅓ oz; 38g) Yoghurt (4 oz; 114 ml)
Fruit and Vegetable	4	Vegetable or fruit (½ cup) eg apple, banana, potato, carrots, cabbage, etc.
Cereal	4	1 slice bread (preferably wholemeal) cereals, rice, macaroni, etc. (1 oz; 28g)

The *meat* group provides protein, iron, thiamine, riboflavin, niacin, phosphorus, zinc and other trace elements.

The *milk* group provides protein, calcium, phosphorus, riboflavin, carbohydrate, fat, minerals and trace elements.

The *vegetable-fruit* group provides fibre, vitamins (especially A and C), minerals and trace elements.

The *cereal* group provides thiamine, protein, iron, niacin, carbohydrate, fibre, minerals and trace elements.

The Cambridge Diet Compared with Other Food

The food guide described above is the one most widely used by dietitians. There have, however, been many criticisms of it. When it was designed, the RDAs for certain nutrients such as phosphorus, iodine, vitamins B-6, B-12, E and K, folic acid, pantothenic acid, biotin and trace elements were not considered. Thus, while an individual can eat the correct number of servings, certain minerals may still be lacking, especially iron. It is a fallacy to suppose that by advising people to 'eat a wide variety of foods' all the requirements will be met, since no one can adequately define 'a wide variety of foods'. Some foods add many calories but no nutrients, others give large amounts of nutrients and few calories. Without a computer it is virtually impossible to choose a wide-ranging selection of food that does contain everything the body needs.

The great advantage of the Cambridge Diet is that it is nutritionally dense and complete. In a small number of calories, every nutrient is included in just the right amounts. This is particularly reassuring to someone who is busy, and does not have the time to work out the nutrient content of a diet from food tables.

CHAPTER FIFTEEN

CAMBRIDGE COCKTAILS

One of the major problems one has to face when going on a diet is boredom. The taste of succulent food is one of the greatest pleasures in life. Strict dieting limits our choice, and the consequent feeling of deprivation we feel is the main reason why most diets fail – we become bored, start to cheat and in no time we are off to the nearest pub or fish and chip shop.

The Cambridge Diet tries to make life easier by providing a variety of appealing flavours. It comes in five milk-shake or cold drink forms – vanilla, chocolate, strawberry, banana and peach – and six hot soup flavours – chicken, asparagus, minestrone, turkey, vegetable and beef. Although I believe that these flavours are very satisfactory and satisfy people most of the time, it is possible to make an almost infinite variety of cocktails using the Cambridge Diet as a base. Most of these variations centre around the use of spices, imitation flavour extracts, artificial sweeteners, diet soda flavours, coffee, curry, tabasco and Worcester sauce. For those on the Diet as sole source, it is most important to use only calorie-free additives, otherwise the object of the diet will be defeated.

Enjoy yourself by letting your imagination run riot. Become an amateur, non-alcoholic, cocktail bar-person. Below I have given some of the recipes devised by Cambridge Counsellors in the United States. For best effect, it is preferable to mix the drinks in an electric mixer, using ice for the cold drinks and hot water for the soups. If you find the drinks not sweet enough, however, then artificial sweetener like aspartame (Canderel) can be used to advantage.

Vanilla Diet

White Russian

1 scoop Vanilla Cambridge Diet
¾ cup cold water
¾ cup loose ice
1½ tsp Instant Decaffeinated Coffee
¼ tsp rum flavouring
¼ tsp brandy flavouring

Lemonade Fizz

1 scoop Vanilla Cambridge Diet
1 cup cold diet lemonade
¾ cup loose ice

Cinnamon Delight

1 scoop Vanilla Cambridge Diet
1 cup cold water
1 cup loose ice
2 dashes cinnamon
¼ tsp vanilla flavouring

Pineapple Crush

1 scoop Vanilla Cambridge Diet
¾ cup cold water
¾ cup loose ice
¼ tsp pineapple flavouring
⅛ tsp banana flavouring
5 drops coconut flavouring

Almond Rum Mocha Cream

1 scoop Vanilla Cambridge Diet
¾ cup water
¾ cup loose ice
¼ tsp chocolate flavouring
¼ tsp almond flavouring
¼ tsp rum flavouring

Hawaiian Cream

1 scoop Vanilla Cambridge Diet
¾ cup cold water
¾ cup loose ice
¼ tsp orange flavouring
⅛ tsp pineapple flavouring
⅛ tsp coconut flavouring

Cambridge Orange Julius

1 scoop Vanilla Cambridge Diet
¾ cup cold water
¾ cup loose ice
¼ tsp orange flavouring

Lemon Cream

1 scoop Vanilla Cambridge Diet
¾ cup cold water
¾ cup loose ice
¼ tsp lemon extract

Grasshopper

1 scoop Vanilla Cambridge Diet
½ cup cold water
¾ cup loose ice
2 drops green food colouring

5 drops mint extract
¼ tsp almond flavouring

Frenched Vanilla

1 scoop Vanilla Cambridge Diet
¾ cup cold water
¾ cup loose ice
⅛ tsp vanilla flavouring
⅛ tsp almond flavouring

Chocolate Diet

Almond à la Roca

1 scoop Chocolate Cambridge Diet
¾ cup cold water
¾ cup loose ice
⅛ tsp almond flavouring
5 drops vanilla flavouring
⅛ tsp coconut flavouring

Cherry Chocolate

1 scoop Chocolate Cambridge Diet
¾ cup cold water
¾ cup loose ice
¼ tsp cherry flavouring

Chocolate Banana Split

½ scoop Chocolate Cambridge Diet
½ scoop Banana Cambridge Diet
¾ cup cold water
¾ cup loose ice
¼ tsp banana flavouring

Hawaiian Fogcutter

1 scoop Chocolate Cambridge Diet
¾ cup cold water
¾ cup loose ice
⅛ tsp chocolate flavouring

Chocolate Mint

1 scoop Chocolate Cambridge Diet
¾ cup cold water
¾ cup loose ice
5 drops mint flavouring

Chocolate Coconut

1 scoop Chocolate Cambridge Diet
¾ cup cold water
¾ cup loose ice
¼ tsp coconut flavouring

Lemon Cream Chocolate

1 scoop Chocolate Cambridge Diet
¾ cup cold water
¾ cup loose ice
¼ tsp lemon extract

Chocolate Cherry Soda

1 scoop Chocolate Cambridge Diet
¾ cup carbonated club soda
1 cup loose ice
⅛ tsp cherry extract

The following recipes can be either HOT or COLD

Jamoca Almond Fudge

1 scoop Chocolate Cambridge Diet
¾ cup HOT or COLD water
1 tsp instant coffee
¼ tsp almond flavouring

Cambridge Cappuccino

1 scoop Chocolate Cambridge Diet
¾ cup HOT or COLD water
1 tsp instant coffee
¼ tsp cinnamon flavouring

Strawberry Diet

Strawberry Pineapple

1 scoop Strawberry Cambridge Diet
1 cup cold water
¼ cup loose ice
¼ tsp pineapple flavouring

Strawberry Delight

1 scoop Strawberry Cambridge Diet
1 cup diet lemonade
¼ tsp coconut flavouring

Passion Fruit

1 scoop Strawberry Cambridge Diet
¾ cup cold water
¾ cup loose ice
⅛ tsp strawberry flavouring
5 drops orange flavouring
5 drops lemon flavouring

⅛ tsp coconut flavouring
⅛ tsp pineapple flavouring
⅛ tsp banana flavouring
⅛ tsp rum flavouring

Bubble Gum

½ scoop Strawberry Cambridge Diet
½ scoop Vanilla Cambridge Diet
¾ cup cold water
¾ cup loose ice
½ tsp orange flavouring
½ tsp cherry flavouring

Tutti Frutti

½ scoop Strawberry Cambridge Diet
½ scoop Banana Cambridge Diet
¾ cup cold water
¾ cup loose ice
½ tsp cherry flavouring
1 tsp vanilla flavouring

Pink Lady

½ scoop Strawberry Cambridge Diet
½ scoop Banana Cambridge Diet
¾ cup cold water
¾ cup loose ice
⅛ tsp strawberry flavouring
¼ tsp coconut flavouring

Super Special

1 scoop Strawberry Cambridge Diet
¾ cup cold water
¾ cup loose ice
½ tsp cinnamon flavouring
¼ tsp almond flavouring

Strawberry Coconut

1 scoop Strawberry Cambridge Diet
¾ cup cold water
¾ cup loose ice
¼ tsp coconut flavouring
¼ tsp vanilla flavouring

Strawberry Daiquiri

1 scoop Strawberry Cambridge Diet
¾ cup cold water
¾ cup loose ice
¼ tsp rum flavouring

Strawberry Fizz

1 scoop Strawberry Cambridge Diet
1 cup diet lemonade
½ cup loose ice

Banana Diet

Banana Frappé

1 scoop Banana Cambridge Diet
1 cup cold water
1 cup loose ice
⅛ tsp coconut flavouring
¼ tsp vanilla flavouring

Creamy Banana

½ scoop Banana Cambridge Diet
½ scoop Vanilla Cambridge Diet
¾ cup cold water
¾ cup loose ice
¼ tsp vanilla flavouring

Tropical Fruit Ice Cream

1 scoop Banana Cambridge Diet
¾ cup cold water
¾ cup loose ice
¼ tsp coconut flavouring
¼ tsp pineapple flavouring
¼ tsp strawberry flavouring
¼ tsp rum flavouring

Banana Nut Milk Shake

1 scoop Banana Cambridge Diet
¾ cup cold water
¾ cup loose ice
1 tsp vanilla flavouring
¼ tsp black walnut flavouring

Banana Nut

1 scoop Banana Cambridge Diet
¾ cup cold water
¾ cup loose ice
¼ tsp black walnut flavouring

Quickie Colada

1 scoop Banana Cambridge Diet
¾ cup cold water
¾ cup loose ice
¼ tsp pineapple flavouring
⅛ tsp coconut flavouring

Hot Banana Cream Pie

1 scoop Banana Cambridge Diet
9 oz (256 ml) HOT water
½ tsp vanilla flavouring

Banana-Orangeade

1 scoop Banana Cambridge Diet
1 cup diet orangeade
½ cup loose ice

Recipes for Cambridge Diet Soups

Celery, mushrooms, spinach, cabbage, carrots, onions
and any other green vegetables may be creatively added
to Cambridge Diet soups. Remember NOT TO BOIL
the Cambridge Diet soup or you risk loss of vitamins.

Cook vegetables separately and after blending the
Cambridge Diet soup, pour over vegetables. You may,
in addition, add a low-sodium bouillon which provides
an excellent broth for added flavour without added salt.
Stir and serve with a sprinkle of Parmesan cheese, dash
of pepper or sprinkle of parsley for added flavour.

The following recipes can be used for either the
Chicken or Beef Cambridge Diet soup:

Cream of Onion Soup

¾ scoop Chicken/Beef Cambridge Diet
¼ scoop Vanilla Cambridge Diet
¾ cup very hot water
1 tsp onion powder
salt substitute & pepper to taste
dash of garlic powder

Cream of Celery Soup

1 scoop Chicken/Beef Cambridge Diet
1½ cup very hot water
1 tsp celery powder
½ tsp parsley flakes
¼ tsp garlic powder
salt substitute & pepper to taste

Curry Soup

1 scoop Chicken/Beef Diet
1¼ cup very hot water
½ tsp curry powder
½ tsp onion powder
5 drops coconut flavouring
dash pepper
dash thyme
½ tsp dried parsley

Double Chicken/Beef Soup

1 scoop Chicken/Beef Diet
1¼ cup very hot water
⅛ tsp poultry seasoning
¼ tsp onion powder
⅛ tsp nutmeg
⅛ tsp garlic powder

Cambridge Diet Soups for Maintenance

Cauliflower Savoury Soup

1 scoop Chicken/Beef Cambridge Diet
1 cup very hot water
1 cup bite-sized cauliflower
1 tbsp chopped onion
⅛ tsp celery seed
Cook cauliflower and onion in the 1 cup of water in a
covered saucepan over medium heat for 5 minutes. Put
1 cup of broth from vegetables mixture (add very hot
water if you need it to make 1 cup) into blender with the
Cambridge Diet and celery seed. Blend on low for 30
seconds. Add vegetables and stir.
CALORIES: 146

Mama's Chicken/Beef Soup

1 scoop Chicken/Beef Cambridge Diet
1½ cup very hot water
½ cup diced celery
¼ cup sliced mushrooms
1 tsp minced onion
¼ tsp herb seasoning
¼ sachet chicken bouillon
Cook celery, mushrooms and onion in small amount of water until tender, approx. 10 minutes. Combine remaining ingredients in blender and blend on low speed for 15 seconds. Stir in cooked vegetables. Garnish with Parmesan cheese, parsley or paprika.
CALORIES: 131

Spicy Rice Soup

1 scoop Chicken/Beef Cambridge Diet
1¼ cup very hot water
⅛ tsp bar-b-cue spice
dash garlic powder
salt substitute & pepper to taste
Combine Cambridge Diet, hot water, and seasoning in blender. Blend on low speed for 10 to 15 seconds. Stir in cooked rice and serve.
CALORIES: 144

Cream of Potato Soup

1 scoop Chicken/Beef Cambridge Diet
1½ cup very hot water
½ boiled potato, peeled and chopped (⅓ cup)
¼ cup cooked, diced celery
1 tbsp minced onion
⅛ tsp substitute salt
dash of pepper
Cut up potato, celery and onion. Boil until tender,

about 10 min. Drain. Put hot water in blender then add Cambridge Diet and remaining spices. Blend on low speed for 10 seconds. Stir in vegetables and serve.
CALORIES: 157

CHAPTER SIXTEEN

CALORIE CONTROLLED RECIPES

This chapter is meant for those people who are on an 'Add-A-Meal Interval' between periods of sole source or on the permanent maintenance plan.

Add-a-Meal Interval

After you have been on the Cambridge Diet sole source for four weeks, you may use the Add-a-Meal dishes of about 400 calories to your three Cambridge Diet meals. You may have one choice from column A, one from column B plus one from column C.

A
5 oz skinless chicken breast
4 oz lean beef mince
4 oz grilled lean beef steak
5 oz white fish
4 oz water-packed tuna fish
4 oz beef liver
3 oz lamb chop
8 oz cottage cheese
3 eggs – omelette or boiled
B
1 cup green beans
1 cup broccoli
1 cup spinach
1 cup carrots

1 cup asparagus
1 cup cauliflower
1 cup cabbage
½ small baked potato
¼ head lettuce and ½ tomato
C
1 slice of whole wheat bread
or 2 slices of diet bread with ½ pat of butter
or 2 tsp of diet margarine

1 oz = 28 g
Use no salt when cooking or use a salt substitute. All meat should be grilled.

Weight Maintenance

The following recipes are included to give you a wider range of calorie-controlled Add-a-Meal for weight maintenance. For most active people, about 1,200 to 1,500 calories, in addition to your Cambridge Diet three times a day, will be ample. Dishes are for one person unless otherwise stated.

Side Dishes – 50 Calories

Relish Plate

1 medium-sized carrot – cut into 12 sticks
1 stalk of celery – cut into 6-9 sticks
3 green onions – 3″×⅜″ (8 cm×1 cm)
10 radishes – ¾″ to 1″ (2 cm to 2.5 cm) diameter

Cauliflower Salad

1 cup thinly sliced raw cauliflower
3 olives, sliced

1 tsp pimento, chopped
1 tbsp vinegar

Mix above ingredients and let stand 1 hour. Serve chilled. If cooked cauliflower is preferred, steam it until tender, then mix with the rest of ingredients and chill. Freshly ground pepper makes a nice addition.

CAULIFLOWER: Eaten as a hot vegetable one may eat 2 cups of flowerets. Steaming is the most nutritious preparation.

Cooked Peas

Cook half a cup of shelled peas in a saucepan with a ¼ cup water, until tender and still green. Drain and season with low-sodium salt to taste. (Peas can also be combined with sliced mushrooms.)

Side Dishes – 100 Calories

Beetroot and Cucumber Salad

¾ cup boiled sliced beetroot
¾ cup raw sliced cucumber
¼ cup plain yoghurt
¼ tsp dill
2 tsp white wine vinegar
1 tsp Dijon mustard

Mix yoghurt, dill, vinegar and mustard together to form a dressing. Pour over sliced beetroot and sliced cucumber and serve.

Baked Apple (serves 4)

(Use 2"; 5cm diameter apples which yield 50 calories each.)
4 2"; 5 cm diameter apples

2 tbsp raisins
Sugar substitute to equal 1 tbsp
pinch of cinnamon
pinch of nutmeg
½ cup unsweetened orange juice

Core apples and fill with a mixture of raisins, nutmeg, cinnamon, and sugar substitute. Pour orange juice over apples. Bake at 350°F (180°C; Mark 4) for 30-40 minutes.

Banana

1 medium banana
sprinkle with sugar substitute
1 pinch of cinnamon

Bake at 350°F (180°C; Mark 4) for 15 to 20 minutes.

Side Dishes – 200 Calories

Tomato Stuffed with Egg and Prawns

Take one large tomato and remove core. Using knife, slightly split tomato in thirds so filling can be mounded in the centre.

Egg and prawns – mix 1 oz (28 g) of prawns with one chopped hard-boiled egg. Add 2 tbsp finely minced green onion and ¼ of a green bell pepper, finely minced. Add 1 tsp Dijon mustard, 1 tbsp plain yoghurt, and salt and pepper to taste. Place in tomato.

Chicken Vegetable Soup (servings for 1 or 4 people)

Serving 1	Serving 4	
2 cups	2 quarts (2¼ l)	chicken stock
¼ cup	1 cup	carrots, diced
¼ cup	1 cup	celery, diced
¼ cup	1 cup	courgettes, diced
¼ cup	1 cup	potato, diced
¼ cup	1 cup	green peas
1 tbsp	4 tbsp	watercress

In a saucepan, combine 2 cups of chicken stock, adding each of the following diced vegetables; carrots, celery, courgettes, potato and green peas. Also add the chopped cress. Simmer slowly until vegetables are tender.

Spinach Salad

2 cups raw spinach leaves
½ cup sliced mushrooms
1 hard-boiled egg – chopped
½ cup boiled, sliced beetroot

Carefully wash spinach leaves. Wash and slice mushrooms. Boil beetroots and chill. Combine all ingredients in bowl, toss and serve.

Spinach Salad Dressing

1 tbsp plain yoghurt
2 tsp red wine vinegar
2 tsp Dijon mustard
pinch of black pepper
few drops of low-calorie sweetener to taste.

Combine ingredients and mix until smooth.

Gourmet Menus – 400 Calories

Lamb Mediterranean (serves 4)

1 lb (454 g) lean lamb leg (trimmed of all fat and cut into 1″ (2.5 cm) cubes and marinaded in Sauce Dijonaise about 1-2 hours).

Sauce Dijonaise
1 small garlic clove
¼ cup Dijon mustard
¼ tsp powdered ginger
½ tsp dried mint
few drops of low-calorie liquid sweetener
1 oz (2 tbsp) white wine

Place on 4 skewers (give each person 4 oz; 113 g meat) and grill about 10 minutes, turning and brushing with remaining marinade.

Rice Pilaf
Bring 1¼ cups (unsalted and no fat) chicken stock, or beef stock, or water to boil, add 1 tbsp minced shallots and ½ cup rice, cover and simmer about 15 to 20 minutes. Then add about 2 tbsp chopped parsley, and low-solium salt to taste. ½ cup of cooked rice per serving.

Dilled Cucumber with Yoghurt (serves 4)
Mix 2 cups of ⅛″ .3 cm) sliced cucumbers with ⅔ cup of plain yoghurt and 1 tsp of dill.

Dessert
One whole orange – approximately 2⅝″ (6.7 cm) in diameter per person.

Breast of Chicken Verde (serves 1 or 4)

1	4	skinned chicken breasts 6-8 oz (170-227 g) each
1 tsp	¼ cup	white wine
¼ cup	1 cup	water
1	2	bay leaves
2	4	whole peppercorns
1 tbsp	¼	mirepoix (chopped celery, carrots and onions)

Delicately poach skinned chicken breasts, breast side down for about 30-40 minutes.

Green Bean Purée (serve over chicken breasts)

4 oz (113g)	1lb (454 g)	green beans
		boiling water – enough to cover beans
		salt (1½ tsp per quart of water)
½ tsp	1 tsp	butter
pinch	pinch	nutmeg

Cut beans into 1″ (2.5 cm) lengths. Boil them uncovered in large pan of boiling salted water until tender (slightly over-cooked). Drain and rinse under cold water. In a food processor or blender purée beans, thin with cooking liquid and reheat in saucepan. Season with butter and nutmeg.

Baked Potato
One whole potato per person. Potato scooped out and mashed with chicken stock and 1 tbsp grated cheddar cheese per person. Season with white pepper and salt. Top with a few grates of cheddar cheese; sprinkle with paprika.

Sliced Tomato
One tomato per person, ¼″ (.64 cm) slices.

Dessert

Purée one medium-sized fresh, ripe, peeled and stoned peach for each person in blender or food processor. Pour purée over half a ripe pear for each person.

Gourmet Dishes – 600 calories

Lamb Stew (serves 1 or 4)

1	4	
6 oz (170 g)	1½ lbs (680 g)	lamb shoulder, in 1″ (2.5 cm) cubes
1 cup	4 cups	beef stock
4 oz (113 g)	1 lb (454 g)	mushrooms, quartered
4 oz (113 g)	1 lb (454 g)	pearl or boiling onions
½ cup	2 cups	haricot beans
1 tbsp	4 tbsp	Dijon mustard
1	4	garlic cloves
½ tsp	2 tsp	rosemary
1 tbsp	4 tbsp	cornflour
2 oz (57 ml)	8 oz (227 ml)	water

Trim off fat and cut the lamb shoulder into bite size (approx. 1″; 2.5 cm) cubes (4 oz; 113 g when cooked). Brown in non-stick cookware. Add beef stock, quartered mushrooms, pearl or boiling onions (peeled), haricot beans, Dijon mustard, finely minced garlic, rosemary, and simmer until onions and haricot beans are tender, about 20-30 minutes. Thicken with cornflour mixed with water.

Marrow

Serve 4 oz (113 g) cooked marrow per person. Steaming is the most nutritious cooking process. Season to taste.

Spinach

Wash and stem spinach and steam until wilted. Season with white pepper and nutmeg and a little salt. Serving size per person is 1 cup of cooked spinach.

Baked Apple

Wash and core 1 or 4 apple(s). Place in baking dish with 1 cup water, a little low-calorie sweetener, plus a clove and a cinnamon stick. Cover and bake in 375°F (190°C; Mark 5) oven for about 30-40 minutes. Pour apricot purée over apples. To purée apricots, peel and stone 3 apricots per person and steam until tender. Purée in blender or food processor.

Butterflied Trout (serves 1 or 4)

1	4	
7 oz (198 g)	1¾ lbs (794 g)	trout, butterflied
2 oz (57 g)	1 cup	fish stock (or use half fish stock and half white wine)
1 small	4	cucumber(s), peeled, seeded and chopped
2 oz (57 g)	8 oz (227 g)	small shrimp
2 oz (57 g)	8 oz (227 g)	crab meat
1 tbsp	4 tbsp	fine herbs or chopped parsley
1 tbsp	4 tbsp	slivered almonds

Trout

To butterfly trout, lay uncooked trout on its side on cutting board. Open the body cavity, inserting knife (belly side) under the backbone and cut through rib bones from head to tail, being careful not to cut through back. Remove backbone and side rib bones. Grill about 4 minutes or pan fry in non-stick cookware about 5 minutes on medium heat. Season with salt and pepper to taste. Top trout with cucumber sauce.

Cucumber/Seafood Sauce

In a saucepan combine fish stock and/or white wine with cucumber (peeled, seeded and chopped), shrimp and crab meat and fine herbs or chopped parsley. (Fine herbs = chopped parsley, chervil, tarragon and chives). Cook until cucumber is tender (about 10 minutes). Serve over trout and sprinkle 1 tbsp almond on top of each serving.

Potato

Cut one medium potato per person in quarters and cook 15-20 minutes in boiling water. When potatoes are tender, drain well. Top with chopped parsley and salt and pepper to taste.

Tomatoes

1 cup small tomatoes peeled per serving. (To peel tomatoes, plunge in boiling water for 10 seconds.) Sprinkle with 1 tsp oregano and heat in non-stick cookware 2-3 minutes.

Marrow

Wash and cut into small pieces, 1 cup marrow per person. Steam until tender. Drain well and season to taste.

Peach

Poach 1 medium-sized peeled peach in 2-3 cups water (or 4 cups for 4 peaches), sweetened with low-calorie sweetener, adding 2-3 cloves, 1 cinnamon stick and a slice of lemon. Poach until tender. Purée 1 cup (or 4 cups) strawberries in blender or food processor, reserving 1 strawberry for garnish on each serving. Pour over peach.

Gourmet Dishes — 800 Calories

Small Chicken with Cherry Sauce (serves 1 or 4)

1	4	
		1 small chicken
1 cup	4 cups	cooking cherries
6 oz (170 ml)	3 cups	chicken stock
1 tbsp	4 tbsp	cornflour

Small chicken
Roast 1 lb (454 g) small chicken at 375°F (190°C; Mark 5) approximately 25-30 minutes. Prick its thigh; when juices run clear bird is cooked.

Cherry sauce
Heat cherries and juice in saucepan with 7 oz (199 ml) chicken stock. When sauce comes to a boil, add 1 tbsp cornflour thoroughly mixed with cold water to thicken. Pour over chicken.

Marrow
One cup marrow per serving. Marrow may be baked or cut up or boiled in a small amount of water. Mash with 1 tbsp butter and season with nutmeg, cinnamon, pepper and salt, if necessary.

Green beans
Wash and string 1 cup of runner beans per serving. Steam until tender. Season to taste.

Tomatoes
Put 1 cup or 4 cups of tomato wedges in a pot and sprinkle with sweet basil, pepper and salt if necessary. Heat through.

Roast Leg of Lamb

One 7-9 lb; 3-4 kg joint serves 16 4 oz; 113 g portions.

To roast, preheat oven to 450°F (230°C; Mark 8). Insert 4-5 cloves of garlic and 1 tbsp whole rosemary under skin of lamb, using pointed knife in 4-5 areas. Place meat on rack, having trimmed as much fat off the outer skin as possible. Roast in 325°F (170°C; Mark 3) oven, 20-25 minutes per lb (454 g) for rare, 25-30 minutes per lb (454 g) for medium and 30-35 minutes per lb (454 g) for well done. Approximate total cooking time should be between 2 and 4 hours. During cooking add 1½ qts (2 l) water, bay leaf, and 4-5 whole peppercorns to create sauce. Remove fat from juice and finish seasoning with a little salt or low sodium salt. Serve 4 oz (113 g) of lamb and ladle 2 oz (57 ml) of au jus (lamb juice) over meat.

For each person serve 1 large roasted potato with or without skin. (Skin is very nutritious.) Slice one red bell pepper and steam until tender. Season with favourite herbs and spices. Steam one cup of sliced courgettes and season.

Fruit salad
For one portion, mix one cup of lettuce, segments of one medium orange, one cup diced pineapple and half cup seedless grapes. Toss with a dressing of 4 oz (114 ml) plain yoghurt mixed with 2 oz (57 ml) of orange juice. Serve chilled.

For the Vegetarian

Vegetarian diet recipes can be equally delicious. If you have been using the Cambridge Diet as your sole source of nutrition, it is a good idea to begin your maintenance programme by using the following recipes. Each meal contains about 250 calories.

For the Add-a-Meal interval, take *two* meals from any of the list of breakfasts, light meals or main meals. This allows you about 500 calories a day, in addition to the 330 calories from the Cambridge Diet.

For weight maintenance, take two or three meals from the list in addition to the three Cambridge Diet meals. The number will depend on whether your weight is stationary or changing.

Vegetarian Dishes

Breakfast – 1

1 oz (28 g) Weetaflakes ⎫
1 oz (28 g) prunes, stoned,
  soaked and chopped   ⎬ (mixed together)
4 oz (114 ml) skimmed milk ⎭
1 average sliced wholemeal toast (1¼ oz; 35 g) topped
  with ¼ oz (7g) cheese spread

Breakfast – 2

2 Ryvitas or wholemeal toast (2½ oz; 71 g) topped
  with ½ oz (14 g) tahini (sesame spread) or ½ oz
  (14 g) low fat spread+1 tsp yeast extract
1 apple (5 oz; 142 g) chopped/grated
½ oz (14 g) dried apricots chopped (soaked together
overnight)
pinch ground ginger
½ oz (14 g) raisins

Breakfast 3

¾ oz (21 g) puffed wheat ⎤
¼ oz (7 g) raisins soaked ⎬ (mixed together)
4 oz (114 ml) skimmed milk ⎦
1 Ryvita topped with 1 banana (6oz; 170 g)
sliced/mashed

Breakfast 4

1 small carton natural yoghurt
1 pear (5 oz; 142 g) cored and chopped
½ oz (14 g) stoned dates chopped
½ oz (14 g) hazelnuts chopped
½ oz (14 g) All Bran
mixed spice/cinnamon to taste

Light Meal – 1

1 wholemeal roll (1½ oz; 43 g) filled with–
1 cooked Vegeburger (grilled, baked, or fried without
oil)
1 tomato, sliced
2 oz (57 g) cucumber, sliced
½ oz (14 g) watercress
1 apple

Light Meal – 2

2 average slices wholemeal toast (2½ oz; 71 g) topped
with–
½ oz (14 g) cheese spread
4 oz (113 g) mushrooms, lightly
poached
2 tomatoes (4 oz; 113 g), halved
and grilled
½ oz (14 g) watercress
1 orange (6 oz; 170 g)

Light Meal — 3

2 average slices wholemeal bread (2½ oz; 71 g) filled
with—
1 oz (30 g) Granose vegetable pâté
½ oz (14 g) watercress
1 tomato, sliced
1 orange

Light Meal — 4

2 average slices wholemeal bread (2½ oz; 71 g) filled
with—
1 banana, mashed ⎤
lemon juice │
¼ oz (7 g) walnuts, chopped ⎬ (mixed together)
½ oz (14 g) watercress ⎦

Main Meal — 1

8 oz (227 g) hot cooked ⎤ mix together, reserv-
  cauliflower, mashed ⎥ ing half cheese for
4 oz (113 g) cottage cheese ⎬ the top; grill
½ spring onion chopped ⎥
seasoning ⎦
4 oz (113 g) fresh/frozen peas, cooked with mint

4 oz (113 g) peaches in fruit ⎤
  juice ⎬ stewed together
2 oz (57 g) raw/frozen ⎥
  raspberries ⎦

Main Meal – 2

4 oz (113 g) cooked potatoes in skins, mashed ⎤
1 oz (28 g) cottage cheese/tofu (soya bean curd) │
½ oz (14 g) spring onions, chopped │ mix together well,
½ oz (14 g hazelnuts, chopped, ground │ form into two
2 tomatoes (4 oz; 113 g), halved and grilled │ burgers and grill/
4 oz (113 g steamed/sautéed cabbage with caraway seeds ⎦ bake or fry without oil

1 pear (5 oz; 142 g), cored and chopped ⎤
2 oz (57 g) raw/frozen blackcurrants ⎦ stewed together

Main Meal – 3

4 oz (113 g) mushrooms, chopped ⎤
4 oz (113 g) beanshoots │
2 oz (57 g) frozen peas │ Stir fry vegetables in
2 tomatoes (4 oz; 113 g) quartered │ the soy sauce and
2 oz (57 g) canned sweetcorn and peppers drained ⎬ either stir in tofu
½ onion finely chopped │ chunks towards the
soy sauce │ end or top with
4 oz (113 g) tofu chunks/ cottage cheese ⎦ cottage cheese

8 oz (227 g) honeydew melon, sprinkled with pinch cinnamon/mixed spice

1 oz (28 g) dried prunes, stoned, soaked ⎤
1 oz (28 g) dried apricots, soaked ⎦ stewed together and puréed

192

1 egg beaten with a little
  water
½ oz (14 g) parsley, chopped   Cook omelette and
2 oz (57 g) canned sweetcorn   fill with seasoned
  and peppers   vegetables
seasoning

4 oz (113 g) fresh/frozen
  peas cooked

1 orange (6 oz; 170 g),
  peeled and its flesh
  chopped
2 oz (57 g) raw/frozen
  blackcurrants

CHAPTER SEVENTEEN

MORE ABOUT EXERCISE

There really is a programme of exercise for everyone who is truly interested in physical fitness. Listed and discussed here are several forms of the most popular exercises available. Specific exercises for the protruding abdomen, thick thighs and legs, toning of slack muscles in upper arms, building up of breasts, or whatever your particular body needs might be, are not included. Should you need special 'toning' exercises you will find many excellent books, articles in magazines and newspapers and literally hundreds of physical fitness centres around the world that can help you tone up where you need it most.

Swimming

I will give most space to swimming, as it is a form of exercise for everyone. So if you can't swim, learn now. Swimming offers some unique opportunities to people who, because of age or disability, have not been able to participate in a physical fitness programme before.

Although swimming can be much less strenuous than many other forms of exercise, the results are just as beneficial in improving cardiovascular and muscular endurance, strength and flexibility.

Swimming will also provide the same psychological benefits that any other physical activity can provide, but for those people who have not been able to experience a positive fitness programme it opens up a new dimension.

Success It provides an opportunity to do something well and to enjoy a feeling of success. This is all too often denied to the person with a disability or of advanced age.

Self Image Being successful at something may enable an individual to enhance his or her self image. A person's regard of self worth and ability may be increased.

Emotional Outlet Swimming is fun, and for persons whose activities are limited, it provides an environment in which frustration may be released safely. To splash, push and kick water is a marvellous release for tension.

Reduced Evidence of Age or Disability Age or physical impairment is far less evident in water. Of those who experience discomfort or inability to walk on land (even those confined to a wheelchair) most will be capable of walking unaided in water. The advantage of buoyancy in water makes possible movement which is impossible on land.

Although special programmes may be needed for individuals with severe problems, many persons are indeed able to participate in a regular swimming programme.

One of my assistants has multiple sclerosis and has, in the past, been in a wheelchair or had to use canes or crutches. When her husband and three of their friends decided to begin the Cambridge Diet and to start a physical fitness programme she was sure she would be unable to participate. They found a local fitness centre that had a pool, and while her husband and friends were pushing weights and walking treadmills she very slowly began water exercises. At the beginning she could only swim half a length of the pool but worked up to 80 full lengths after about two months. Being able to participate in something not only helped her achieve better physical fitness, but also allowed her the opportunity of being included in the group.

Swimming has long been a part of rehabilitation programmes and is now widely used as a relatively painless and yet total physical fitness exercise.

Jogging and Running

One has only to look out of the window at some time during the day to observe at least one or two joggers.

Jogging has become very popular and I am a keen devotee of it myself. In fact I was one of the first to begin jogging in Cambridge. Back in 1960 I could be seen jogging along Gog Magog Hills in Cambridge and was even interviewed by a Cambridge newspaper and photographed. I was considered something of a freak. Times have changed!

Those who are physically and mentally up to this form of activity are totally exhilarated by it and converted to it. If, however, you are extremely overweight your body has to be conditioned beforehand, otherwise it can be very dangerous and precipitate a heart attack.

This is why it is most important to see your doctor before taking up jogging. The king of jogging, Jim Fixx, who wrote *The Complete Book of Running*, died of a coronary attack while jogging at the age of fifty-two. Although he advised other people to see a doctor regularly, he never did himself.

Also, jogging can cause other problems. Apparently doctors' surgeries are full of joggers with tendonitis, inflamed or ruptured Achilles tendon caused by repeated running uphill, sore shins, fractures, and blisters by the thousand.

To help avoid trouble do not wear tight T-shirts which can cause 'jogger's nipple', get a good pair of shoes, and stick to grass at first.

How do you start a jogging programme? SLOWLY! Take it easy at first, running slowly for 5 minutes, then walk for the same time and repeat until you are comfortably tired. As you become conditioned and the weeks roll by, you can begin to run faster and extend the time, but never attempt more than you feel you can cope with. If you are really interested, consult one of the many books on this form of exercise for a good programme of action. Adopt a running style and have plenty of determination.

Is it worth it? Those who have mastered this form of exercise are extremely enthusiastic and almost fanatical in their praise of it, so much so they become evangelical. They feel a sensible running programme is the *best* way to keep heart and lungs in good condition.

Gym Exercises and Weight Lifting

Judging by the large number of people who are joining health and fitness centres, strenuous gym exercises and weight lifting seem to fit the need of many people.

While many will feel it is too strenuous, people who exercise in gyms regularly do develop very efficient cardiovascular systems. The benefits are obvious — having excellent muscle tone, a highly efficient heart, and stronger lungs. Weight lifting is not an aerobic exercise but nevertheless it will build those extra muscles needed to increase your metabolism.

Modern gyms now have trampolines which, besides providing aerobic exercise, are especially beneficial for overweight people, because they alleviate the problem of landing on the ground with too much force. Mini-trampolines are also available for those who want to use one in the privacy of their own homes.

Rather surprisingly, working out every day will not give as good results as every other day, especially over a long period of time. All weight-training activities should be supervised by trained personnel, who can ensure strict observance of procedure to prevent injury and see that you obtain maximum benefit.

Exercise Machines

All fitness centres and gyms are equipped with a myriad of exercise machines giving a whole range of body-trimming exercises for the really enthusiastic body builder. For the person who prefers to do his or her exercising in the privacy of home, there are now many types of multi-gym exercise machines. These used to be obtainable only with expensive, weight-operated equipment. The modern machines, however, are compact and designed to high standards, making them suitable for home use.

Different types of exercises that can be done on these machines include: overhead pulls, bench press, shoulder press, rowing, squats and upper torso curls. Also, for those people who find cycling outdoors too dangerous, there are stationary cycling machines for home use.

Aerobic Dancing

Ordinary dancing is fun, and aerobic dancing is too! Aerobic dancing is a combination of exercise and dancing and is a complete physical fitness programme. This is your opportunity to express yourself physically to music by laughing, yelling, jumping, kicking, jogging, stretching, sliding and swinging.

Judging by the overflowing classes that are springing

up everywhere, aerobic dancing has become an over-night sensation for women. And although aerobic dancing classes are quite popular it is not necessary to join a class to enjoy its benefits. No great skill or technique is required. There are literally hundreds of books, tapes and records to help you learn it at home. I would suggest that to begin the programme, you seek expert advice, and start very slowly. To reap full benefit, aerobic dancing should be done a minimum of three times weekly.

The dedicated aerobic dancer will tell you that it is never boring because it can be varied and integrated with other aerobic activities. Also, it has the potential of helping develop grace, poise and rhythm. For this reason people are able to stay in the programme longer.

Aerobic dancing, if implemented properly and practised and supervised according to the rule books, is thought to lessen the chances of developing coronary heart disease or related vascular ailments.

Bicycling

Bicycling is unique among popular fitness programmes in that it does *not* take weeks for a beginner to build up a gradual exercise plan.

If, however, you have previously been a sedentary person, a little sensible caution is advisable. For those over the age of thirty-five and who are a bit out of shape, or those who suffer from a heart, lung or circulatory disease, it would be best to see a physician to determine your level of fitness before starting.

Most of us have grown up as cyclists but gave it up after leaving school. Cars and sitting in front of television sets have greatly affected this once totally normal form of exercise.

As a boy growing up in East Anglia I travelled extensively all over Europe, often cycling over 100 (161 km) miles a day. Lack of time and my hectic schedule have almost put a complete stop to the cycling I am able to do. However, I still do hire a bicycle on occasion and find it just as exhilarating an activity as ever.

Cycling is a marvellous way to attain a heart rate that expands the blood flow to the muscles and increases the lung's capacity to absorb oxygen, thus avoiding heart and lung disease.

So much is offered to the cyclist; freedom to exercise whenever the urge strikes, an opportunity to get out into fresh air, and economical transportation.

I would give just one caution about cycling: learn how to ride safely. Obtain a manual of bicycle safety rules and become a sensible, safe cyclist. Not every city has the same problem that exists here in Cambridge (20,000 students and 19,000 of them use cycles), but an irresponsible cyclist runs the risk of not living long enough to reach the goal of being physically fit!

Walking

It has been said that walking is the safest and most efficient form of exercise. Merely increasing the amount of daily walking can give great benefits. You actually do *not* need to worry about technique or exercise regimen – just wear comfortable shoes and begin the walking habit.

I have long been accused by my family and friends of walking them to exhaustion! I enjoy walking and walking with speed and vigour and I personally find walking most efficient for improving overall fitness. It uses more muscles in a continuous uniform action than most other forms of exercise and it remains accessible to you throughout your lifetime.

Walking has become the most often used medical programme to prevent heart related diseases and to rehabilitate those who have been stricken with heart trouble.

There are approximately four basic forms used in walking programmes:

Strolling The slowest form of walking, but just as significant in results. After dinner strolls or walking the dog, Sunday strolls, all can begin with 20 minutes a day and be stretched into two, three and four hours. The miles begin to add up to a significant amount of work.

With strolling you find the repetitious movements of the body's walking-muscle groups aid circulation and helps to burn off some calories (at a very slow rate, of course).

Normal Walking Normal walking is usually considered an average speed of three mph, and can be used as a fitness programme simply by doing more of it. How? Walk to work. Take the stairs instead of the lift. Drive or bus to within a mile of your destination and walk the rest of the way. Walk to a colleague's office instead of phoning. During coffee/tea breaks take a walk, stretch your legs. Walk before and after meals, if for only 15 minutes. During inclement weather, walk inside a shopping mall. This can be most convenient in hot humid weather as well as snow and cold. A walk before a meal can actually DEPRESS your appetite and help you control your eating and ultimately your weight. It can even stimulate your thinking processes by increasing oxygen in the brain.

Aerobic Walking This is any style of walking done with speed. It consists of sustained rapid breathing while vigorously moving your arms and legs for at least fifteen minutes – up to thirty minutes, three times per week. Just maintain a brisk pace. As you become more physically fit you can speed up and extend your time, helping to continue making progress.

Long Distance Walking This is for people who really enjoy walking and are physically fit.

To help the long distance walker, there are now many long distance routes mapped out and illustrated in guidebooks for you to choose. Once you feel ready for it, try it!!

To Exercise or Not

Having read this chapter may have made you so physically tired that any thoughts of taking up exercise may have already evaporated. But do consider it carefully. The benefits are the joy of being physically fit and healthy, and having a new and lower set-point. You will find it easier to keep those newly lost pounds off.Whatever you take up, it is important that you enjoy it! So re-read this chapter and decide to experiment and find out for yourself what type of exercise you think you would like doing best. In the long term you will only persist if it gives you pleasure.

CHAPTER EIGHTEEN

QUESTIONS AND ANSWERS

Here is a list of the most frequent questions asked about the Cambridge Diet, and my answers to them.

1 **Q.** Will I feel hungry when on the Diet?

   A. Some hunger is experienced during the first one or two days but on the third day it usually disappears completely. This is because your body has adjusted to its new balance of receiving only 330 calories per day.

   Should you cheat, you will become very hungry indeed. Eating food only stimulates your hunger more, so it is best to stick to the Diet and do not supplement it, at least for four weeks when you can have a break.

2 **Q.** Will everybody lose weight on the Cambridge Diet?

   A. Yes, the only difference is how much and how fast. Men burn more calories than women, therefore men will lose weight more quickly.

3 **Q.** Can people have an unlimited amount of diet soft drinks while taking the Cambridge Diet as a sole source of nutrition?

   A. Diet soft drinks should be limited. Many diet drinks contain sodium, which, if consumed in excess may cause the body to retain water and slow the weight loss process. Some diet soft drinks also contain caffeine, which may have a stimulant or irritant effect on the body.

4 **Q.** Why is it recommended that the Cambridge Diet be used as a sole source of nutrition for no more than four consecutive weeks?

  A. When the doctors who participated in the clinical trials were asked what was the maximum time they would recommend the diet be used sole source, without medical supervision, the consensus of opinion was four weeks.

5 **Q.** Does the Cambridge Diet contain enough protein when taken as a sole source of nutrition?

  A. The 8½ years of research developing the Cambridge Diet concluded that 33 grams of protein per day, in combination with 44 grams of carbohydrate provide sufficient protein to maintain the lean body tissue required.

6 **Q.** How much water should I drink when on the Cambridge Diet?

  A. It is very important to consume at least eight glasses of water or other liquid per day. Since our bodies consist of over 60 per cent water, it is very important that we constantly replace our body fluids. Sufficient liquid intake is also necessary to maintain proper kidney function.

7 **Q.** Is it necessary to take additional vitamins while on the Cambridge Diet?

  A. Providing you take at least three scoops of Cambridge Diet per day there is no necessity for additional vitamins, unless prescribed by your doctor.

8 **Q.** I find that although I am faithful to my diet my weight loss levels off from time to time. Why is this?

   A. This is known as 'plateauing' and is very natural. Plateaus can have any number of causes. For instance, it is normal for females to plateau before menstruation, but this is fluid retention and is temporary. Often, just a little snack here and there adds enough calories to sustain the body and eliminate further weight loss. Diet sodas generally contain a high amount of salt, and an excess of diet soda can cause plateauing.

9 **Q.** Once you arrive at your goal, how do you maintain your weight?

   A. If a person achieves a desired weight and then goes back to the bad food habits of a lifetime that put the weight on in the first place, it is inevitable that the weight lost will be regained.

   The Cambridge Diet gives rapid weight loss, but it also provides a sound nutritional base for those who are at their desired weight and who want to keep it. The method I recommend is that you will take your Cambridge Diet three times per day even when your desired weight is achieved. Along with this nutritional base you should then add one or two meals totalling 400 to 800 calories until the scales show how many calories you can absorb and still maintain your desired weight.

10 **Q.** I weigh 110 lbs (50 kg) and maintain my trim figure by eating very little. I often tire easily and I wonder if I am getting proper nutrition?

   A. Thousands of people who look trim are actually suffering from poor nutrition. They tire easily and have few energy reserves. Most of them subsist without breakfast and have very little nutritious food throughout the day. By taking the Cambridge Diet drinks three times per day along with a balanced meal, they feel altogether different. Their energy level is much higher and they are obviously in much better health.

11 **Q.** Is alcohol allowed while taking the Cambridge Diet as a sole source of nutrition?
   A. No. Alcohol contains seven calories per gram and is of no other significant nutritional value.

12 **Q.** Is it all right to drink coffee while taking the Cambridge Diet as a sole source of nutrition?
   A. Consumption of large quantities of coffee or Colas is not recommended. If you feel you must drink them, the decaffeinated forms are preferred. Caffeine acts as a stimulant to the body systems and sometimes provides an irritant effect. Herbal teas offer a pleasant alternative.

13 **Q.** What is the shelf life of the Cambridge Diet?
   A. Recommended shelf life for the Cambridge Diet is two years unopened; 3 or 4 months opened, but sealed with the plastic lid.
   Certain nutrients are rapidly oxidized when in contact with light, air and heat. The most harmful effects to the product can come from leaving the lid off the can.

14 **Q.** Some days I feel completely satisfied with only two Cambridge Diet meals. Do I need to take the third meal?
   A. Yes. Three Cambridge Diet meals provide all the necessary nutrients for one day to keep your body in a good nutritional state.

15 **Q.** If I am really hungry, can I take a fourth Cambridge Diet meal without spoiling my diet?

A. Some people may require additional energy for their activities, such as those involved in heavy physical work and strenuous athletics. An extra Cambridge Diet meal may be necessary to provide extra energy in balanced form.

16 **Q.** At what age should a person refrain from taking the Cambridge Diet?

A. A person who has medical problems should not be on any type of diet without a doctor's supervision. However, the Cambridge Diet Plan has helped extremely elderly people who have a problem with eating sufficient food to provide proper nutriton.

17 **Q.** Why does the label on the Cambridge Diet say that it should not be taken by children?

A. Children under the age of twelve should not be on any drastically reduced calorie diet without being under a doctor's supervision. Since Cambridge Diet is nothing more than food and vitamins, there is no reason why children cannot take the Cambridge Diet as a food supplement for nutritional purposes.

18 **Q.** Why are women who are pregnant or breast feeding advised not to use the Cambridge Diet?

A. Pregnant and lactating women can use the Cambridge Diet as a nutritional supplement but not as their sole source of nutrition, because they may need more nutrients than other people.

19 **Q.** Do you recommend exercise with the Cambridge Diet?

A. Do not start a strenuous exercise programme at

207

the same time as you start the Cambridge Diet.
(If you are already taking exercise then you
may continue it.) Moderate exercise is useful
once you start to lose weight, providing that it is
approached with caution and not done with
excess. Walking or cycling is excellent exercise,
but start slowly, and do not overdo it at the
beginning.

20 **Q.** How can the Cambridge Diet help athletes?
  A. It provides a very good nutritional foundation
  for athletes whose performance is largely
  dependent upon their bodies receiving the
  precise balance of nutrients which the
  Cambridge Diet provides.

21 **Q.** Will the Cambridge Diet bring on ketosis?
  A. The Cambridge Diet is specifically formulated
  with 44 grams of carbohydrates in addition to
  the protein and fat present. This combination
  produces a mild ketosis which can be a benefit
  to those on weight loss programmes as it gives a
  slight euphoric effect while somewhat curbing
  the appetite.

22 **Q.** Does the Cambridge Diet have any effect on
  menstrual cycle?
  A. Rapid weight loss with very low calorie diets
  may temporarily affect the menstrual cycle
  patterns; ovulation, however, is not inter-
  rupted. This cycle is usually corrected within a
  few months, as body metabolism adjusts.

23 **Q.** After the second day on the Cambridge Diet I
  suffered a severe headache. Why is this?
  A. Occasionally, during the initial three days a
  person may experience carbohydrate withdrawal and may develop a headache. This is a

temporary effect and should be tolerated. A simple tablet for headaches, for example aspirin, taken for a day or two will improve the problem.

24 Q. Just after starting on the Cambridge Diet I suffered from diarrhoea. Is this normal?

A. This is a minor problem and is considered a possible transient effect that will last for only a short time. Some people have systems that are not used to the mineral content in the Cambridge Diet. The solutions are very simple. One is to take a bulk laxative such as Metamucil, or Fibrogel. This will provide bulk to the intestinal system and alleviate the problem. Another is to consume a full glass of water following the Cambridge Diet meal in order to dilute the effect of the minerals on the body. A third solution is to take the Cambridge Diet in the form of mini meals (six half portions per day) initially to slow the mineral intake.

Another possible cause of continued diarrhoea is lactose intolerance. Some people cannot digest the lactose in milk products, and diarrhoea can occur. If this is the case, an addition of the enzyme lactase is sufficient to solve the problem. Lactase is available from chemists or health food stores and is a very inexpensive solution to the problem.

25 Q. I experience a feeling of euphoria on the Cambridge Diet. Is this normal?

A. This is very normal and should not cause any concern. In fact, why not just enjoy it!

26 Q. I am under treatment for depression. Is it safe for me to take the Cambridge diet?

A. There is nothing in the Cambridge Diet plan

that would interfere with depression therapy. It is important, however, that any diet you undergo be supervised very carefully by your doctor or psychiatrist.

27 Q. I find that I am having trouble getting my usual amount of sleep. Why is this?

A. It is not uncommon for a person to require less sleep when their body is put in proper nutritional balance. I know of many cases where people thought that they require 9 or 10 hours of sleep per night, only to find that when they lost weight and maintained nutritional balance their sleep requirement dropped considerably. Having an extra hour or two awake each day may be a pleasant side effect of the Cambridge Diet.

28 Q. I feel thirsty sometimes. Is this normal?

A. It is normal to experience thirst on occasion when dieting. The solution is simple. Drink more liquids. At least eight glasses of liquid should be consumed each day in addition to the Cambridge Meals.

29 Q. I seem to have a recurring problem with heartburn and have an ulcer. Will the Cambridge Diet aggravate this condition?

A. On the contrary, the Cambridge Diet is easily digested, and reports indicate that it has a very soothing effect on the stomach. Some people swear that the Cambridge Diet drinks have reduced their symptoms drastically. It may be necessary to take six mini meals per day instead of the three regular Cambridge Diet meals, but the ingredients in the Cambridge Diet will not interfere with ulcers or ulcer medication. If you are on medication for ulcers, be sure to contact your doctor before going on any diet.

30 **Q.** I notice a tendency towards bad breath for the first few days. Why is this?

A. A mild ketosis may develop when on the Cambridge Diet as your sole source of nutrition and this may affect your breath slightly. Simply brush your teeth more often, and use mouth wash, sugar-free chewing gum or breath fresheners.

31 **Q.** I found shortly after starting on the Cambridge Diet that I was constipated. Is this normal?

A. The Cambridge Diet contains sufficient roughage for most people. When one goes on any diet including the Cambridge Diet, much less bulk is being consumed, and therefore there is much less bulk to be eliminated. As a result, bowel movements are much less frequent. This is normal, and should not cause immediate concern. When the body is ready, the bowels will move. If physical discomfort is actually being suffered then a natural laxative such as Metamucil or Fybogel should be taken according to instructions.

32 **Q.** Whenever I start on the Cambridge Diet plan I feel nauseated. Is this normal?

A. On occasion a person's body will be upset by the minerals present in the Cambridge Diet. This is usually very short lived. The benefits of the Diet far outweigh any short-term discomfort and should be tolerated. Usually, a full glass of water following your Cambridge meal will eliminate this problem. If it still persists, start taking your Cambridge Diet along with a regular meal. Another solution is to break the

Cambridge Diet down into six mini meals per day, and follow each meal with a glass of water to dilute the effect of the minerals.

33 **Q.** I noticed that I felt dizzy a few days after starting on the Cambridge Diet.

A. Dizziness is a possible transient effect of any diet and should only last for a day or so. It is most often caused by the diuretic effect that accompanies any low calorie diet. During the first few days of the Diet, the body will give up a considerable amount of water, which reduces the amount of fluid circulating in the body. This can be compensated for by drinking large volumes of liquid and avoiding quick changes in position or extreme exertion during the first few days of the Diet.

34 **Q.** I have already had one heart attack. Can I take the Cambridge Diet?

A. Check with your doctor before going on any diet. The Cambridge Diet is low in cholesterol, low in sodium and low in fat. It is recommended by most heart specialists.

35 **Q.** I have had surgery for cancer. Can I take the Cambridge Diet?

A. There are no contra indications in using the Cambridge Diet. Scientists are looking closely at the relationship between cancer and proper nutrition, but you should check with your doctor before using the Diet.

36 **Q.** Can people with high blood pressure take the Cambridge Diet for weight loss and is it permissible to take diuretics?

A. Many people with high blood pressure have experienced extremely positive results taking the Cambridge Diet for weight loss. Not only has there been a significant drop in blood pressure, but also a normalization which allowed a decrease in medication previously required. It is very important that these people consult their doctors, especially if they are taking medication. The Cambridge Diet, taken as a sole source of nutrition, will itself cause water loss. Any artificial diuretics added to the diet could seriously deplete your potassium balance and cause dizziness, weakness and fatigue. For this reason, medication having a diuretic effect should not be taken concurrently with the Cambridge Diet except with the approval of a doctor.

37 **Q.** I am on a low sodium diet. How much salt is there in Cambridge?

A. The Cambridge Diet contains approximately 500 mg of sodium per serving, or approximately 1,500 mg salt per day. A doctor should be consulted if the dieter has been placed on a low sodium diet, to make sure that the sodium intake is not in excess of the doctor's recommendation.

38 **Q.** I have a thyroid condition and am on medication. Can I safely take the Cambridge Diet?

A. The Cambridge Diet is compatible with all standard thyroid procedures, but I would recommend consulting your doctor before starting any diet.

39 **Q.** Can a person with diabetes be on the Cambridge Diet?

A. Many of my colleagues have found that by changing from three Cambridge Diet meals per day, to six mini meals the dieter's caloric intake is controlled. We have seen great success with diabetic patients using the Cambridge Diet. Diabetics are cautioned, however, not to embark on any diet programme without first consulting their physician.

40 **Q.** How does the Cambridge Diet affect those with hypoglycemia?

A. Hypoglycemia is the opposite of diabetes. Low blood sugar often results from poor nutriton. The Cambridge Diet made into six mini meals per day does an excellent job of keeping the blood sugar level in hypoglycemic people.

41 **Q.** I have a tendency towards gout. Can I use the Cambridge Diet?

A. The Cambridge Diet, because of the balance of its low protein and carbohydrate content, should not cause much of an increase in the uric acid content of the body. It is advisable, however, for a gout-prone person to work closely with a doctor so that the uric acid content can be monitored, and medication prescribed if necessary. Individuals who lose a considerable amount of weight generally show reduced uric acid levels and are generally less prone to gout attack.

APPENDIX 1

Composition of the Cambridge Diet

A	Servings	g
	Meal size	34
	Three meals/day	103

B	Macronutrients	Per day	% RDA
	Calories	330	NA
	Protein	33	75
	Carbohydrate	44	*
	Fat	3	100
	Fibre (indigestible carbohydrate)		*

* RDA not established

C	Micronutrients	Per day mg	% RDA (USA)
	Vitamin A	1	100
	Thiamine	1.5	100
	Riboflavin	1.7	100
	Niacin (Nicotinamide)	18	100
	Pyridoxine	0.1	100
	Pantothenic acid	5	100
	Biotin	0.2	100
	Folic acid	0.4	100
	Vitamin B^{12}	0.003	100
	Vitamin C	60	100
	Vitamin D	0.01	100
	Vitamin E	10	100
	Vitamin K	0.067	100

Calcium	800	100
Phosphorus	800	100
Magnesium	350	100
Potassium	2010	**
Sodium	1500	**
Chloride	1800	**
Iron	18	100
Zinc	15	100
Iodine	150	100
Copper	2	**
Manganese	4	**
Selenium	0.06	**
Molybdenum	0.150	**
Chromium	0.06	**

** US RDA has not been established but the Food and Nutrition Board of the National Research Council recommends these quantities as being within the range required.

D	*Typical list of ingredients (UK formulation)*	
	Ascorbic acid	Magnesium oxide
	Alpha-tocopherol acetate	Manganese sulphate
	Aspartame	Monocalcium phosphate
	Biotin	Nicotinamide
	Calcium pantothenate	Phytonadione
	Carrageenan	Potassium chloride
	Cholecalciferol	Potassium molybdate
	Chromic sulphate	Pyridoxine hydrochloride
	Colouring	Riboflavin
	Copper sulphate	Sodium citrate
	Cyanocobolamine	Sodium selenate
	Ferrous fumarate	Soya flour
	Flavouring	Thiamine hydrochloride
	Folic acid	Vitamin A acetate
	Lecithin	Xanthan gum
	Low fat milk powder	Zinc oxide

APPENDIX 2

Height and Weight Tables
Desirable weights (in indoor clothing)
MEN   MEN
of Ages 25 and Over   of Ages 25 and Over

Height (with shoes on) 1 inch heels		Weight (lbs)			Height (with shoes on) 2.5cm heels	Weight (kg)		
ft	ins	small frame	medium frame	large frame	(cm)	small frame	medium frame	large frame
5	2	112-120	118-129	126-141	157.5	50.5-54.5	53.5-58.5	57.0-64.0
5	3	115-123	121-133	129-144	160	52.0-56.0	55.0-61.0	58.5-65.0
5	4	118-126	124-136	132-148	162.5	53.5-57.0	56.0-62.0	60.0-67.0
5	5	121-129	127-139	135-152	165	55.0-58.5	57.5-63.0	61.0-69.0
5	6	124-133	130-143	138-156	167.5	56.0-60.0	58.5-65.0	62.5-71.0
5	7	128-137	134-147	142-161	170	58.0-62.0	56.0-66.5	64.5-73.0
5	8	132-141	138-152	147-166	172.5	60.0-64.0	62.5-69.0	66.5-75.0
5	9	136-145	142-156	151-170	175	62.0-66.0	64.5-71.0	68.5-77.0
5	10	140-150	146-160	155-174	177.5	63.5-68.0	66.0-72.5	70.0-79.0
5	11	144-154	150-165	159-179	180	65.0-70.0	68.0-75.0	72.0-81.0
6	0	148-158	154-170	164-184	183	67.0-71.5	70.0-77.0	74.0-83.5
6	1	152-162	158-175	168-189	185.5	69.0-73.5	71.5-79.0	76.0-85.5
6	2	156-167	162-180	173-194	188	71.0-76.0	73.5-81.5	78.5-88.0
6	3	160-171	167-185	178-199	190.5	72.5-77.5	76.0-79.0	80.5-90.5
6	4	164-175	172-190	182-204	193	74.0-79.0	78.0-86.0	82.5-92.5

WOMEN
of Ages 25 and Over

WOMEN
of Ages 25 and Over

Height (with shoes on) 2 inch heels		Weight (lbs)			Height (with shoes on) 5 cm heels (cm)	Weight (kg)		
ft	ins	small frame	medium frame	large frame		small frame	medium frame	large frame
4	10	92-98	96-107	104-119	147.5	42.0-44.5	43.5-48.5	47.0-54.0
4	11	94-101	98-110	106-122	150	42.5-46.0	44.5-50.0	48.0-55.0
5	0	96-104	101-113	109-125	152.5	43.5-47.0	46.0-51.0	49.5-56.5
5	1	99-107	104-116	112-128	155	45.0-48.5	47.0-52.5	51.0-58.0
5	2	102-110	107-119	115-131	157.5	46.5-50.0	48.5-54.0	52.0-59.5
5	3	105-113	110-122	118-134	160	47.5-51.0	50.0-55.0	53.5-61.0
5	4	108-116	113-126	121-138	162.5	49.0-52.5	51.0-57.0	55.0-62.0
5	5	111-119	116-130	125-142	165	50.5-54.0	52.5-58.5	57.0-64.5
5	6	114-123	120-135	129-146	167.5	52.0-56.0	54.5-61.0	58.5-66.0
5	7	118-127	124-139	133-150	170	53.5-57.5	56.0-63.0	60.0-68.0
5	8	122-131	128-143	137-154	172.5	55.0-59.5	58.0-65.0	62.0-70.0
5	9	126-135	132-147	141-158	175	57.0-61.0	60.0-66.5	64.0-71.5
5	10	130-140	136-151	145-163	177.5	58.5-63.5	62.0-68.5	66.0-74.0
5	11	134-144	140-155	149-168	180	61.0-65.0	63.5-70.0	67.5-76.0
6	0	139-148	144-159	153-173	183	63.0-67.0	65.0-72.0	69.5-78.5

For girls between 18 and 25, subtract 1 lb (454 g) for each year under 25.
(Courtesy of Metropolitan Life Insurance Co.)

BIBLIOGRAPHY

Books on the Cambridge Diet

Birch, R.D., *The Cambridge Diet: Medically speaking*, 1982, Hexi Publishing, P.O. Box 560, Sandy, UT 84091.
Blanton, B., Goldstein, J.M., Silverman, A., *The Cambridge Diet Psychologically Speaking*, 1983, Breakthrough Publishing, Washington.
Boe, E., *The Official Cambridge Diet Book*, 1983, Bantam Books, New York.
Ignasias, Sheila and Dennis, *Recipes for use with the Internationally acclaimed Cambridge Diet Plan*, 1983, Slim-lines Publications, Salisbury, Maryland 21801.
Wilson, F.C., *The Cambridge Miracle*, Atlantis Publishing of Palm Beach Inc., P.O. Box 2096, Boca Reton, Fl. 33432.

Other Books

Batten, Jack, *The Complete Jogger*, 1977, Harcourt Brace Jovanovitch, New York.
Blackburn, G.L. and Bray, G.A. Editors
Management of Obesity by Severe Calorie Restriction. The symposium on very low calorie diets, held June 3-6 1983, Falmouth, Massachusetts. PSG Publishing Co., Inc., Massachusetts 01460
Cannon, G. and Einzis, H., *Dieting Makes you Fat*, 1983, Century Publishing, London.
Cooper, Kenneth H., M.D., *The Aerobics Program for Total Well-Being*, 1982, M. Evans, New York.

Cooper, Mildred and Kenneth H., M.D., M.P.H., *Aerobics for Women*, 1972, Bantam Books, New York.

Editors of Consumer Guide, *The Running Book*, 1978, Beekman House, New York.

Katz, Jane, with Bruning, Nancy P., *Swimming for Total Fitness*, 1981, Dolphin Books/Doubleday, Garden City.

Kuntzleman, Charles T. and the Editors of Consumer Guide, *The Complete Book of Exercise*, 1979, G.K. Hall, Boston, Mass.

Parr, Richard B., Ed. D., Bachman, David C., M.D., Bates, H. Noble, M.D., *The Diet that Lets you Cheat*, 1983, Crown, New York.

Sloane, Eugene A., *The All New Complete Book of Bicycling*, 1980, Simon & Schuster, New York.

Sorensen, Jacki with Burns, Bill, *Aerobic Dancing*, 1979, Rawson, Wade Publishers, Inc., New York.

Stuart, R.B., and Davis, B., *Slim Chance in a Fat World: Behavioral Control of Obesity*, 1972, Research Press, Champaign.

Swank, R.L. and Pullen, M.H., *The Multiple Sclerosis Diet Book*, 1972, Doubleday, New York.

Swartz, B., *Diets Don't Work!*, 1982, Breakthrough Publishing, Houston, Texas.

U.S. American National Red Cross, *Swimming and Water Safety*, 1968, Textbook, Washington.

U.S. American National Red Cross, *Adapted Aquatics (Swimming for Persons with Physical Impairments)*, 1977, Doubleday, Garden City.

Walford, R.L., *Maximum Life Span*, 1983, W. W. Norton, New York.

Yanker, Gary D., *Walk Your Way to Health and Fitness*, condensed from *The Complete Book of Exercisewalking*, Readers Digest, June 1984, p. 141, Readers Digest Association, Inc., Pleasantville, N.Y.

Articles

Cook, R.F., Howard, A.N., and Mills, I.H., 'Low-dose mianserin as adjuvant therapy in obese patients treated by a very low calorie diet', *International Journal of Obesity*, 5, 1981, pp. 267-72.

DiBiase, G., Mattioli, P.L., Contaldo, F. and Mancini, M. 'A very low calorie formula diet (Cambridge Diet) for the treatment of diabetic-obese patients', *International Journal of Obesity*, 5, 1981, pp. 319-24.

Grant, A.M., Edwards, O.M., Howard, A.N., Challand, G., Wraight, E.P. and Mills, I.H., 'Thyroidal hormone metabolism in obesity during semi-starvation', *Clinical Endocrinology*, 9, 1978, pp. 227-31.

Hickey, N., Daly, L., Bourke, G. and Mulcahy, R, 'Outpatient treatment of obesity with a very low calorie formula diet', *International Journal of Obesity*, 5, 1981, pp. 227-30.

Howard, A.N., 'Dietary treatment of obesity', in *Obesity: Its Pathogenesis and Management*, edited by Silverstone, T., 1975, Medical and Technical Publishing Co., pp. 123-54.

Howard, A.N. 'The treatment of obesity by starvation and semi-starvation', in *The Treatment of Obesity*, edited by Munro, J.F., 1979, MTP Press, pp. 139-64.

Howard, A.N. 'Possible complications of long-term dietary treatment of obesity', in *Proceedings of Serono Symposium*, edited by Mancini, M., Lewis, B., and Contaldo, F., 1979, Academic Press, London, pp. 349-63.

Howard, A.N. and McLean Baird, I., 'The long term treatment of obesity by low calorie semi-synthetic formula diets', IX International Congress of Nutrition, Mexico, 1972.

Howard, A.N. and McLean Baird, I., 'The treatment of obesity by low calorie diets containing amino acids', *Nutrition and Dietetics*, 1973.

Howard, A.N. and McLean Baird, I., 'The treatment of obesity by low calorie semi-synthetic diets', in *Recent*

Advances in Obesity Research: 1., edited by Howard A.N., 1974, Newman Publishing, pp. 270-3.

Howard, A.N. and McLean Baird, I., 'Very low calorie semi-synthetic diets in the treatment of obesity. An inpatient/outpatient study', *Nutr. Metab.*, 21, 1977, pp. 59-61.

Howard, A.N., and McLean Baird, I., 'A long-term evaluation of very low calorie semisynthetic diets: an inpatient/outpatient study with egg albumin as the protein source', *International Journal of Obesity*, 1, 1977, pp. 63-78.

Howard, A.N., Grant, A., Edwards, O., Littlewood, E.R. and McLean Baird, I., 'The treatment of obesity with a very low calorie liquid-formula diet: an inpatient/outpatient comparison using skimmed-milk protein as the chief protein source', *International Journal of Obesity*, 2, 1978, pp. 321-32.

Howard, A.N., Grant, A., Challand, G., Wraight, E.P. and Edwards, O., 'Thyroid metabolism in obese subjects after a very low calorie diet', 1977, Second International Congress on Obesity.

Howard, A.N., Grant, A., Challand, G., Wraight, E.P. and Edwards, O., 'Thyroid metabolism in obese subjects after a very low calorie diet', *International Journal of Obesity*, 2, 1978, p. 391.

Howard, A.N., 'The historical development, efficacy and safety of very low calorie diets', *International Journal of Obesity*, 5, 1981, pp. 195-208.

Howard, A.N., and McLean Baird, I., 'Physiopathology of protein metabolism in relation to very low calorie regimens', in *Recent Advances in Obesity Research: III*, 1981, John Libbey & Co., London.

Howard, A.N., 'The Cambridge Diet: A response to criticism', *J. Obesity and Weight Regulation*, 3, 1984, pp. 65-84.

Kreitzman, S.N. 'Low Calorie Formulated Foods for Weight Reduction'. *Cereal Foods World*, 30, 1985, pp. 845-7

Kreitzman, S.N., Pedersen, M., Budell, W., Nichols, D., Krissman, P. and Clements, M., 'Safety and Effectiveness of Weight Reduction Using a Very-Low-Calorie Formulated Food', *Arch. Intern. Med.*, 144, 1984, pp. 747-50.

Krotkiewski, M., Toss, L., Björntorp, P. and Holm, G., 'The effect of a very low calorie diet with and without chronic exercise on thyroid and sex hormones, plasma proteins, oxygen uptake, insulin and c peptide concentrations in obese women', *International Journal of Obesity*, 5, 1981, pp. 287-93.

Lamberts, S.W.J., Visser, T.J., and Wilson, J.H.P., 'The influence of caloric restrictions on serum prolactin', *International Journal of Obesity*, 3, 1979, pp. 75-81.

McLean Baird, I., Parsons, R.L. and Howard, A.N., 'Clinical and metabolic studies of chemically defined diets in the management of obesity', *Metabolism*, 23, 1974, pp. 645-57.

McLean Baird, I., and Howard, A.N., 'A double-blind trial of mazindol using a very low calorie formula diet', *International Journal of Obesity*, 1, 1977, pp. 271-8.

McLean Baird, E., Littlewood, I.R. and Howard, A.N., 'Faecal transit time and nitrogen balance in patients receiving a new low calorie formula diet', 1977, Second International Congress on Obesity.

McLean Baird, I., Littlewood, E.R. and Howard, A.N., 'Safety of very low calorie diets', *International Journal of Obesity*, 3, 1979, 399.

McLean Baird, I., 'Low calorie formula diets – are they safe?' *International Journal of Obesity*, k5 1981, pp. 249-56.

Moore, R., Grant, A.M., Howard, A.N., and Mills, I.H., 'Treatment of Obesity with triiodothyronine and a very-low-calorie liquid formula diet', *The Lancet*, Feb. 2, 1980, pp. 223-6.

Moore, R., Grant., A.M., Howard, A.N., Mehrishi, J.N., and Mills, I.H., 'Changes in thyroid hormone levels, kinetics and cell receptors in obese patients treated with T₃ and a very low calorie formula diet', in *Recent Advances in Clinical Nutrition*, 1981, J. Libbey & Co., London.

Moore, R., Mehrishi, J.N., Verdoorn, C. and Mills, I.H., 'The role of T₃ and its receptor in efficient metabolisers receiving very low calorie diets', *International Journal of Obesity 5*, 1981, pp. 283-96.

Scheaffer, Henry R.R., Olefsky, J.M. 'Glycemic Effects of Intensive Calorie Restriction and 180 Calorie Refeeding in Non-Insulin Dependent Diabetics'. *J. Clin. Endo. and Metab.*, 61, pp. 917-25

Shapiro, H.J., 'Report of a comparative study: a new very low calorie formula diet versus a conventional diet in the treatment of obesity', *International Journal of Obesity*, 2, 1978, p. 392.

Trott, D.C. and Tyler, F.H., 'Evaluation of the Cambridge Diet. A New Very-Low-Calorie Liquid-Formula Diet', *Western Journal of Medicine*, 30, no. 1, 1981, pp. 18-20.

Visser, T.J., Lamberts, S.W.J., Wilson, J.H.P., Docter, R. and Hennemann, G., 'Serum Thyroid Hormone Concentrations During Prolonged Reduction of Dietary Intake', *Metabolism*, vol. 27, no. 4, 1978, pp. 405-9.

Wilson, J.H.P. and Lamberts, S.W.J., 'Nitrogen balance in obese patients receiving a very low calorie liquid formula diet', *American Journal of Clinical Nutrition*, 32, 1979, pp. 1612-16.

Wilson, J.H.P. and Lamberts, W.J., 'The effect of triiodothyronine on weight loss and nitrogen balance of obese patients on a very low calorie liquid formula diet', *International Journal of Obesity*, 5, 1981, pp. 279-82.

Wilson, J.H.P., and Lamberts, S.W.J., 'The effect of obesity and drastic caloric restriction on serum prolactin and thyroid stimulating hormone', *International Journal of Obesity*, 5, 1981, pp. 275-8.